Moments

That

Matter

Finding the Grace in

Living, Dying, and Surviving Loss

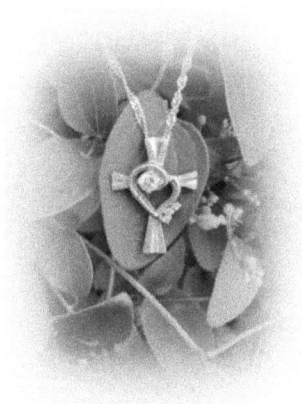

Though sorrow may enter my heart,

There will always be room for love.

By

Diane Fasselius

Contents

Dedication ii

About the Author v

Preface.. vii

Introduction – A Story 1

Part I: The Power of Stories.................................. 5

Part II: Health Care Choices 197

Part III: What Does Dying Look Like?............... 216

Part IV: Spirituality... 244

Part V: Epilogue.. 260

Part VI: Selected Bibliography and Further Reading 263

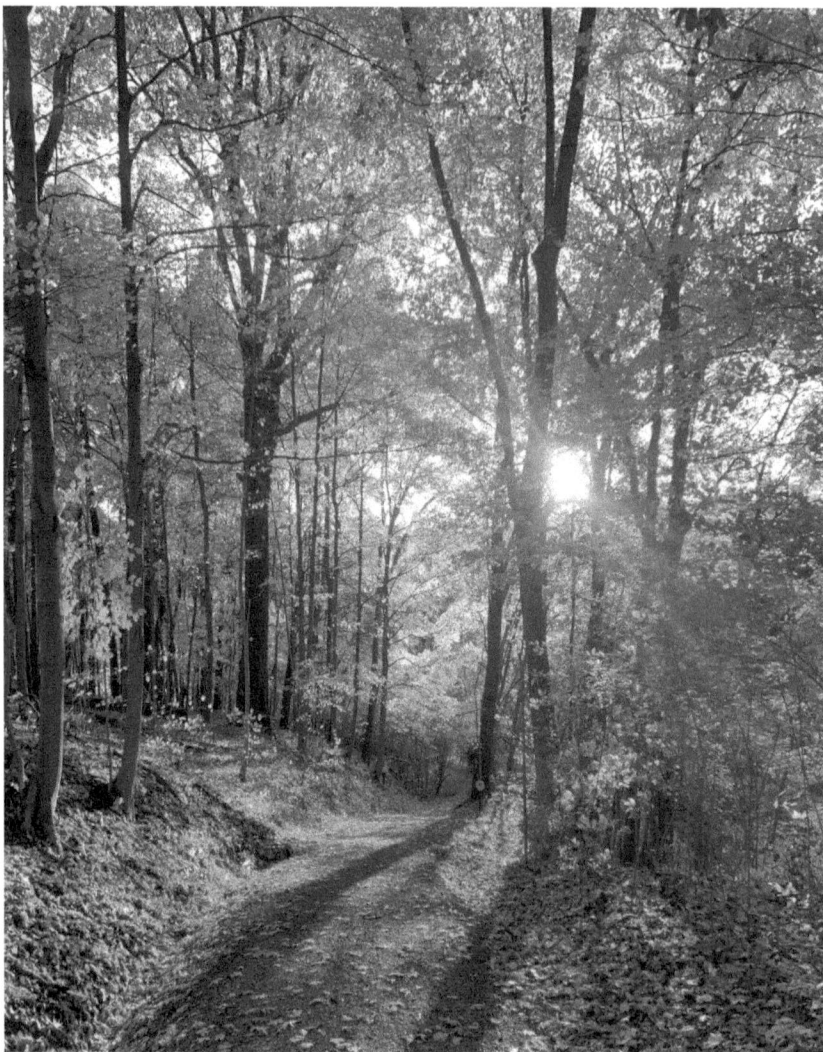

No matter the falling of the leaves or the winding of the road, the sun is always there beckoning us forward.

Dedication

This book is dedicated to the people who have been the greatest influence in my life.

First would be my parents. They not only gave me life and taught me how to treasure it, but they taught me respect, honesty, integrity, truth, and much more. Many times without words. They gave me the grounding that has sustained me throughout life. I am forever grateful for the firm foundation of living they taught by role-modeling for me how to live. No one's life is perfect, and even through imperfections, I was given many life lessons. Through their lives, they taught me how to not only live and celebrate the good times but also how to survive through tough times. It's interesting how we don't recognize the impact people have on our lives until we are older and even more so when they are no longer with us. I miss you, Mom and Dad, I will love you always, and I thank God every day that you were my mom and dad.

Next, I want to recognize my husband, John, the man with whom I shared life for what seems like a very short time on this earth. He taught me more about living than I could ever have imagined. To him, I am forever grateful for helping me grow a grateful, happy, and humorous heart. I will love him forever and beyond, and I can't wait until we meet again.

I would not be writing this if it were not for the boys who call me Mom, Mommy, and Mother. My three sons. I humorously refer to my three sons as my very own "Three Wise Guys." I have always been grateful for the miracle of these boys in my life. When we become parents, we don't realize how much we will learn from our children, but they have taught me some of the most important lessons in life. No words could ever explain how much I love them or how grateful I am to them for giving me so many lessons and blessings in life.

My oldest son once commented, "In my next life, I'm not having parents, they're too hard to raise." In reality, they really have raised me to be a better person. Thank you, boys. I love each of you more than life itself. I wouldn't be the person I am today without each of you polishing my rough edges to become a better person. You have challenged me in many ways to become a better human being. I hope I have risen to the challenge. Thank you.

I have also been privileged in life to have many friends and co-workers who have helped shape me into a more virtuous person. Their influence has been profound as they supported me and encouraged me throughout much of my life, coming and going at just the right time when I needed them. Life brings many blessings, and family and friends are some of the greatest gifts we receive.

Thank you to those mentioned above, but also to each and every person I have been privileged to encounter throughout this wonderful life. We cannot help but be touched and impacted by everyone we meet in this life. Each and every one of you has left an imprint upon my heart that carries your name and can never be erased. My heart is more beautiful because of you.

"Some people come into our lives and quickly go. Some stay for a while, leave footprints on our hearts, and we are never, ever the same".

— Flavia Weedn

About the Author

The author has worked in Health Care as a nurse for over 40 years. She started her nursing career after working in clerical positions for 9 nine years, and then went back to school and spent years intermittently going to school to obtain her nursing degree. Her lifelong desire has been to keep learning every day. Through her nursing experience, she found one of the most rewarding aspects of nursing was helping patients better understand their particular health situation.

Knowledge is power and helping others to attain that knowledge and understanding about their health, whatever it is they need to know, has become one of her passions. From personal experience, she believes it is part of each of our life's mission to help others along their way in life and hopefully find some humor and fun along the way. Working with chronic illness and in hospice has helped her appreciate the importance of offering whatever we can to make another's day the best it can be. Nursing has allowed her the privilege of being a witness to some of the most kind, courageous, resilient, and grateful people in this world.

Her husband died at a young age, leaving her to raise three young children. Having experienced health care "from the other side of the bed," and challenged to find the courage and motivation to continue to live life despite the challenges confronting her, she eventually went on to accomplish a BA degree in Psychology and Religious Studies. It seemed fitting for the next part of her professional journey to include hospice work.

This book was inspired in an effort to help health care workers, professionals, people interested in exploring End of Life issues, families facing illness, friends who want to help others, and anyone challenged to be making decisions about health care choices and advance directives. Good choices can only be made when all the information is available with explanations about potential outcomes of those choices.

Preface

"Never question the truth of what you fail to understand,
for the world is filled with wonders."

L. Frank Baum, <u>Rinkitink in Oz</u>

Unless a person learns this truth, he/she runs the risk of getting paralyzed by life's pain and disappointments and may never fully experience the true joy and happiness this sacred life has to offer. The life we are privileged to live truly is a mystery.

A dear friend once shared an inspirational quote from Soren Kierkegaard, "Life is not a problem to be solved, but a mystery to be lived." It can be hard to comprehend the meaning of that statement until we have many years of living behind us and we find ourselves "lost" on a wayward portion of the road we never anticipated. A place where we find ourselves fully "lost" in the mystery of life.

Years of experience have proven it's good to have plans, but one can't always expect those plans to work out the way one had hoped. Like a road to any destination, there can be many twists and turns that are not expected. We eventually get to the destination following the path of our choosing. That path may be smooth and straight or rugged and crooked. We start out with a destination in mind but never really know where the path will lead or what we will encounter on the path. This may not be the place we thought we'd be, and it may not be the place we want to be, but it becomes a place where we find ourselves. And for each of us, it is best if we can figure out how to navigate the path, however unforeseen or unwanted it may be.

It is a certain, if not consistent, theme in life that we will experience some form of loss. Events that put us on a detour in our path. We may not know how or when it will happen, but it is certain to happen. The gift may well be not knowing how or when those event(s) may occur. There usually is little or no control over the specifics of the event or events that put us on this detour from our planned route in life. We then have to re-navigate the map for the life we will live.

This journey of mystery, called life, often brings many unknowns and circumstances we would prefer not to encounter. Sometimes, we find ourselves off the road, on the shoulder, down a path that seems to lead to nowhere. We have to navigate the potholes and the bad surfaces as well as cross over unwanted bridges, through deep valleys, and over mountainous terrain. We may not know for sure where the path will lead or what we will encounter. The smooth path is seldom the one that lasts forever. There is rarely a clear map to lead us through these off-road experiences. There seems to be no instructions for the detour, and no assured way to navigate an alternate route. But that doesn't eliminate the unavoidable necessity that we must continue on. It is also worth mentioning that sometimes those "detours" do bring unexpected blessings and "gifts" we might never have anticipated.

As a hospice nurse, I have encountered many people who are on that "detour" part of their journey. No one plans to be dealing with a terminal illness or a limited number of days on their journey in life. But it happens every day to many people. The people who are served in hospice are all on a detour. This isn't what they had anticipated for their life. It is here on those detours that we find some of the most wonderful and beautiful stories of survival and witness the GPS recalculation of their life's journey. These people experience all kinds of struggles in finding their way. They have to embrace the unknown and confront the idea of not being on their hoped-for, planned, straight, narrow, and smooth path. They are confronted with the challenge of making this unexpected path as smooth, straight, and tolerable as possible. Their stories are hope-filled, inspiring, sad, and often filled with heartache. But there is also love, hope, comfort, joy, and even some peace in their stories.

Megan McKenna shares a beautiful reflection in her book, And Morning Came, when she tells about the "great violinist Itzhak Perlman whose braces attest to his childhood battle against polio. Once on a New York stage, in the middle of a performance, one of his four violin strings snapped. The orchestra stopped, the audience gasped, and the conductor dropped his baton. But Perlman signaled him to go on, and he finished the entire piece, brilliantly transposing the music to accommodate the remaining three strings. Afterward, he told the audience that this 'has been my vocation, my lifelong mission to make music out of what remains'."

Making music out of what remains is what we all hope to do. Making music from what remains of our lives, our loves and dreams, our hopes and fears, our sufferings and deaths, our struggles and our faithfulness, our communities and relationships after we lose a loved one."

The following pages contain stories of hope, disappointment, courage, and faithfulness. There are stories of kindness and goodness and stories that reveal some of the greatest human virtues in this world. They will show the impact that compassion and love have on the ability to lessen pain and to heal the hurting heart. These stories show how human nature, in its most basic and innocent form, has the great power to transform that which may seem intolerable or unbearable. These are stories of holding the hurting heart in the warmth of a blanket of love and compassion. Unable to change the destination, there is so much to offer to make the journey less painful.

Working in the field of chronic illness and end-of-life has taught me so much. Life is one of the most profound teachers we have if we are open to learning from what we experience. It may not be the arena of education we anticipated or the lesson we wanted to learn, but there is meaning and wisdom from all of life if we choose to be open to the lesson. The Dalai Lama has said, "When you lose, don't lose the lesson."

As a nurse working with chronic illness and the dying, it seems one of the most beautiful and often avoided options in health care for end-of-life is hospice care. I hope the information in this book will help dispel some of the deep-seated fears about dying, death, and hospice care. I hope there may be a story or two that resonates with the reader and might offer some music of hope to help make the detour of life a little easier when one of the strings that provided the music is broken. I hope for comfort for the reader if they are struggling to find their way on an unfamiliar path. Hopefully, some measure of enjoyment can be found in the music of life that remains, and one can learn how to sing again when grappling with loss and struggling to travel harmoniously along this mysterious journey of life.

The stories that follow are all intended to be anonymous. Names have been changed, and although some of the situations may sound familiar, there is no intention to violate anyone's privacy or anonymity in the sharing of these stories. They are offered in an innocent effort to share the challenges others have faced on their path to the end of life and provide hope for the reader that no one ever needs to feel alone in their struggles to make meaning out of the broken music of their life. We all share the common thread of struggling and suffering in life and especially when facing the challenges of a limited number of days.

A framed message from Mother Teresa sits on my desk at the hospice office and reminds me daily,

"I feel like a pencil in God's Hand.... God writes through us..... and however imperfect instruments we may be.... he writes beautifully."

- Mother Teresa

God bless all of you and thank you for taking the time to read these pages.

Introduction – A Story

A mother camel and her baby camel were having a conversation. The baby camel said, "Mother, why do we have such big hooves for feet?" The mother camel replied, "You see, we have these big three-toed hooves, so when we are trekking across the desert, we don't sink into the sand, and we can walk easier." "Oh, OK," said the baby camel. "Well, then, why do we have these long bushy eyebrows?" Again, the mother camel answered, "We have these thick, long, bushy eyebrows to keep the blowing sand out of our eyes so we can see where we are going." Then the baby camel asked, "Well, what about these big humps we have on our backs. Why do we have those?" So the mother camel explained, "You see because the desert is dry and can be a long way to cross, we have those humps to store the extra water we need to make the journey." The baby camel seemed somewhat appeased with the answers but still looked confused and a little puzzled and had one more question. So he said to the mother camel, "I understand about the big three-toed hooves to keep us from sinking into the sand as we walk, and it makes sense that our big bushy eyebrows help keep the sand from our eyes so we can see where we are going. I also understand why we need the humps on our backs to carry the extra water we need for the long journey across the dry, hot desert." "But there is something I still don't understand." "Well, what is it?" asked the mother camel. The baby camel replied, "Well, then, why are we here in the Omaha Zoo?"

That can be a very daunting question. How did I get here? And what am I supposed to do here? I don't believe there is an all-encompassing answer to that question. Each person must discover for themselves what it is that will make sense of the life where they find themselves. The darkness we feel when we have experienced a deep loss leaves us overwhelmed, trying to figure out how to continue on with life. Nothing will ever be the same. Nothing is normal anymore. We have no energy, no ambition, and hope seems out of reach. What do we do? How do we go about understanding this situation, and how do we make sense of the turmoil that now defines our life?

There is hope in knowing that others have also experienced something similar. No two people experience loss or the death of a loved one in exactly the same way. But there is some relief and support in knowing others have been on a similar path. There is a benefit in knowing others have survived something similar. The benefit of support from others who have gone through something similar can be helpful and provide some meaning and encouragement to continue on despite feeling so very lost at the moment.

My hope is that the stories that follow will provide a sense of comfort, knowing others have walked the same sand-laden desert of loss. Maybe the stories will be the thick three-toed hooves that help someone from sinking deeply into the sands of despair. Maybe the information shared will help keep our eyes clear to see there is a path through the windblown sands of loss. Or maybe there will be moments of recognizing those places of oasis needed to nourish the thirst for life still hidden deeply within us.

It is my hope these stories will support, encourage, and hopefully nourish and sustain the reader who may feel lost in the foreign land of loss and grief, which seems to have no road map or any sense of direction to a better place. May there be a gentle encouragement to live the life given to us, despite the circumstances where we find ourselves.

If you are reading this, you, too, may have a story to share. Someone may need to hear your story, and everyone needs to tell their story. I hope this inspires the reader to be open to sharing their story and letting others become part of the healing. There is great wisdom in understanding the healing that comes with telling our story. There is healing in being able to keep telling our story until we no longer need to tell our story.

Along with the stories, you will find inspirational quotes to hold in your heart, music lyrics that might resonate with you, and other spiritual supports that may be helpful. I offer my deepest condolences for any loss you hold deeply in your heart and also sincere support and prayers for every effort and struggle as you encounter the challenge of returning to a full life. The victory is in the living. The honor is in living fully as you embrace the gift of the loved one who still lives on in your heart and your memory.

Being unable to pick up and go on from loss, no matter how great or small, is to give in to the power of that loss and thereby let it take control. In many ways, it can destroy some of the most important parts of your life. Don't let that happen.

"The best way out is always through."

Robert Frost.

"I believe that no matter what 'plot' each of our stories may follow, deep down we all want one thing. We want our lives to matter. We want our stories to be of significance. Nobody wants to feel like the world wouldn't miss him if he'd never lived....." John C. Maxwell from "Your Life Can Be a Great Story."

Like the baby camel, there may be a very good reason you're in "Omaha," even if it doesn't make sense.

Part I: The Power of Stories

What is so great about a story? Well, in truth, everything. Stories connect us. And a good story has power. The power to energize, motivate, influence, entertain, teach, support, soothe, to make us feel something we might never have discovered if we had not heard the story. Stories do so many things. Stories help to propel us beyond ourselves. They are the connective tissue of the human race. As children, we yearned to have stories told to us. We never cared what the story was about. We just loved stories without realizing the impact they could have on us.

"The shortest distance between two people is a story."

Terrence Gargiuio

Stories create the bridge between one mind and another. They can create a connection from one heart to another. Stories are at the very heart of being human and give insight into where we are from, where we are currently, and where we are heading. Stories can give meaning to our past experiences and create a stronger memory of our history. A good story will make us feel something and make us care. It creates that connection we all desperately long for in life. "I want to hear your story" conveys a message of "I care enough about you to want to know more about you." "You matter to me."

Storytelling becomes even more important for those who have experienced loss. Whether the loss resulted in finding a new path in life, coping with illness, learning to live without someone who was loved dearly, maybe finding a more meaningful job, rebuilding a home, or just finding hope in the deep seat of our soul, stories help clarify, redefine and bring meaning to what has happened. Stories help our souls begin anew, to breathe fully and deeply after loss. Stories help us feel deeper compassion for others who have trod a path similar to our own. There is hope and healing in knowing others have walked a similar path of heartache. Sharing our story helps us see beyond the heartache. Stories help us grow out from underneath the hardened surface of the hurtful part of our journey. We cannot wish heartache and sadness away until we have woven them into the fabric of our lives. Stories create the threads that are woven into the tapestry of life to create the beautiful masterpiece it was intended to be.

Telling and retelling our stories can transform our life experiences and give meaning to the pain we have endured. Telling our story also helps release us from the imprisonment that enslaves us to the pain of loss. Stories can be medicine for the spirit and healing for the soul. The power of a story is limitless.

When we experience a life-changing event like the death of a loved one, there is a strong desire to understand how this event fits into our life. How could this have happened to me? What did I do to contribute to this pain in my life? What does this mean for me now and for the unknown and frightening future ahead of me? My life story now needs to be re-written. I am no longer on the path I planned for or hoped to be on. How do I make sense of this senseless event in my life? Why am I in this "zoo" part of my life?

Healing starts with telling your story. It can start anywhere. Every part of your story is important. Every story is unique and unlike any other. It will unfold in the pattern and way it is supposed to. We just need to have the courage to start telling the story. It can become the most significant strategy for finding the meaning of the situation. Your story needs to be told, and it also needs to be heard.

In hospice work, it is a privilege to work with people who are in the final phases of their life. It is a privilege to enter into their life story at a time when they are most vulnerable. They are hurting and feeling lost in a world and life that seems to have betrayed them with a terminal or life-limiting illness. The finish line, their destination, and the conclusion to their story are within sight. How does one write this final chapter, this final paragraph, or this final sentence of their life? The sense of hopelessness at this time can feel overwhelming. How can the conclusion to their story be anything but bad? Those who work in hospice care know better. This final phase of life can be so much more than just an ending. We all know how we anticipate the ending of things. We eagerly await the finish of a class, a semester, a race, or childhood in favor of becoming an adult, the end of a pregnancy when we are blessed with the miracle of birth. We all know how we eagerly anticipate the ending of a good book.

Life is no different. The ending can be filled with experiences and opportunities that offer learning, insight, and meaning into things we may never have thought about. It can bring opportunities to offer and receive love and forgiveness. The potential for growth at the end of life is limitless. It's all about choices. There are always choices in life: give up, give in, or give it all you've got.

As we daily unwrap the gift of life, we may be unaware that it just might be that the best has been saved until last.

"Save the Best for Last" By Vanessa Williams

Sometimes the snow comes down in June

Sometimes the sun goes 'round the moon

I see the passion in your eyes

Sometimes it's all a big surprise

'Cause there was a time when all I did was wish

You'd tell me this was love

It's not the way I hoped or how I planned

But somehow it's enough

And now we're standing face to face

Isn't this world a crazy place

Just when I thought our chance had passed

You go and save the best for last

Sometimes the very thing you're looking for

Is the one thing you can't see

Sometimes the snow comes down in June

Sometimes the sun goes 'round the moon

Just when I thought our chance had passed

You go and save the best for last

Songwriters: Phil Galdston / Jon Lind / Wendy Waldman-Parker

Stories of Moments that Matter

In hospice work, we meet people from every walk of life. Death has no preference for age and is impartial to all. Hospice cares for infants who have just entered the world, as well as centenarians. Hospice workers meet people where they are in life with respect for who they are, where they've been, their life stories, and the relationships they have in life. There is no judgment, and the agenda and expectations belong to the person being served in hospice care. Hospice workers come into the person's life to serve them and offer the best chance at adding the best last chapter to their life story.

There are those who don't fully understand how or why those who work with someone facing death find the work so special.

"What Would Ever Possess You To Want To Do A Job Like This?"

I really don't remember how I answered Mary's question that day, or if I did at all! I have thought of that question many times. What exactly would possess a person to want to be a hospice aide? I have to agree; it certainly doesn't sound like a very glamorous job by any means. But there is so much more to it than showers, backrubs, and lotioning.

Herb was getting weaker every time I visited him. As I helped Herb walk to his recliner, his steps became slower. He became short of breath and needed to rest. His shower was finished, and it had exhausted him terribly. Now, he rested comfortably in his recliner, positioned by the window "to keep an eye on things". As I bent down to remove the gait belt from around his waist, he looked directly into my eyes and patted my arm. "Thanks so much! I feel like a new person", he said.

If only Mary could have heard that, I thought. That might have answered her question.

Sharon wasn't that much older than me. I so enjoyed seeing her each week. She was a proud wife, mother, and grandmother. Even on a not-so-good day, she made chocolate chip cookies and sent them to her granddaughters. She was so proud of those kids, always talking about their accomplishments. After her bath, I would set her hair in rollers. She had beautiful hair that curled easily. We created a beauty shop atmosphere as we talked about different things. I enjoyed pampering her with a bath and doing her hair and nails. Once, Sharon told me, "You provide the very thing that makes the biggest difference and gets the least recognition". All women love pampering and looking pretty.

If only Mary could have known Sharon. That might have given her a little more insight.

Last week I helped Jim with his shower. Dementia had taken his short-term memory. Jim was still able to perform most of his care but needed constant cueing. I stood behind, watching as he looked in the mirror and combed his gray, thinning hair. Suddenly I could see what Jim saw in the mirror. I saw a good-looking young man, full of energy, with his whole life ahead of him. With one hand, Jim combed a full head of thick, dark hair. With the other hand, Jim pressed a perfect wave across the top of his head. He took the bottle of Old Spice and poured a bit into his hands, rubbed them together, and patted them on his face and neck. Standing up straight and tall, he adjusted his collar and looked in the mirror. Turning his head from side to side, he sized up the handsome man from both angles. A broad smile of satisfaction crossed Jim's face. He was ready for a Saturday night date with his favorite girl. For that brief moment, dementia had no hold on Jim.

Oh, I wish Mary would have been standing beside me looking in that mirror too.

Caitlin was a very beautiful girl with dark eyes and long black hair, and she was only 26 years old. Her dreams and future plans were rearranged by her cancer diagnosis. Everything was changing. Caitlin tried so hard to remain strong and "resilient," as she called it. She knew her deteriorating condition was bringing sadness to her family as the Christmas holiday approached. Despite her efforts, she became weaker and needed more help. On one of my visits to see her, Caitlin asked me to comb her long, beautiful hair. I told her she looked like a Christmas Angel. She laughed as she looked at her choice of clothing for the day. "Do they wear sweats and a T-shirt?" I assured her I thought they did and that angels look beautiful in anything they choose to wear. The last day I saw Caitlin, I gently applied lotion to her soft skin. I was glad she was peaceful and not in any pain. She was so tired. Knowing she could still hear me, I told her she would always be my Christmas Angel. Slowly, she opened her eyes and looked at me. With a soft whisper, she said, "Thank you", and closed her eyes again. Caitlin died a few hours later. On earth, we cried, but Heaven rejoiced. They welcomed their newest Christmas Angel.

O, how I wish Mary could have known Caitlin. She would have been touched by this Angel, too!

It's difficult to put into words exactly "what possesses me to want to do a job like this", as Mary put it. Hospice aides develop a unique connection with their patients. We share their excitement over new grand-babies and listen because they still have something to say. We guide an unsure step, lighten situations with humor and reassure a confused mind. Hospice Aides feel the incredible warmth of hugs from frail arms and see the unspoken words of gratitude in grateful eyes. We get teary-eyed when patients promise to watch over us from Heaven, and our hearts ache when they die.

Being a hospice aide has so many rewards. I get back so much more than I could ever give. Aren't I the lucky one?

Oh, Mary! If only you knew!!!

(Hospice aide)

"Not all of us can do great things, but we can do small things with great love…"

- Mother Teresa

In Your Eyes

You smiled and welcomed me into your home. I could see the uncertainty in your eyes. Here, a complete stranger, coming to take care of you, doing something you had done for yourself for years. I saw the sadness in your eyes as you talked about the difficulty of not only accepting help but also the reality of knowing you did need help.

As we talked, a friendship quickly formed, and the conversation became easy. I began to see the softness in your eyes as you recalled memories of your younger days, telling me about your parents and grandparents. Your eyes danced as you told of your childhood antics. The stories made me laugh, and I could see the sparkle in your eyes as you remembered those carefree days.

Your eyes told beautiful stories. I saw the love in your eyes as you talked about meeting "that special girl" at the Melody Mill dance hall and how you both loved to dance the night away. I could see the tenderness in your eyes when you glanced her way. Now 65 years later, she's still your special girl.

A father's pride showed in your eyes when you spoke of your children and grandchildren, so very proud of their talent and accomplishments. I thought your heart would burst as you spoke of the newest great-grandchild that recently joined your family. Each child had a special place in your heart, and your love for them was so strong and evident. Your stories made me feel like I knew each one of them personally. You excitedly told me about those who had stopped by recently or those who were on their way home to see you soon. Your eyes danced with laughter when you told about loading up the whole family in a bus for a fun-filled vacation across the country camping, fishing on the Mississippi, and the fish fry dinners you hosted for family and friends. Everyone was always welcome, and no one left hungry. The memories were priceless, and the stories and laughs were abundant.

Childlike satisfaction showed in your eyes as you enjoyed a glass of root beer. Your hospitality never missed a beat, always asking if there was anything I would like. It was more satisfying to see you enjoy that root beer. Sadness showed in your eyes as you spoke of special family and friends no longer living and how much they meant to you. I saw the tears well up in your eyes as you remembered the horrors of war. With each visit to your home, you always welcomed me with a smile that warmed my heart. I so enjoyed coming to see you. You never failed to let me see the genuine gratitude in your eyes as you thanked me for helping you. With each visit, I could see your slow, gradual decline as ordinary tasks became more difficult. I could see the fear and awareness in your eyes as you realized you were getting weaker. The end was getting near. Although you were tired, you seemed determined to hold on until you knew all was well and your loved ones were in the right place. I saw the unspoken goodbyes in your eyes. I knew, and you did too. I think the red cardinal outside your window knew too. I saw him pause for a short time. Was that a quick thank you for seed and friendship before he flew on ahead to announce your impending arrival? Your eyes became tired and so heavy, unable to fight the inevitable.   Sometimes this job just plain hurts. I'd be lying if I said my heart didn't ache as I drove away from your home that last day. With tears spilling from my eyes, I realized how truly fortunate I am.

I have been given an unexpected gift, not one all wrapped with shiny ribbons, but instead a unique gift that brings purpose and meaning to my life. You and your friendship were gifts to me. You touched my heart and made me a better person.

I know God smiled and welcomed you into his home too.

(Hospice aide)

"Look Who's Here"

There she sat, this fragile but spunky little nun, in her recliner in her room at the convent where she shared life with her congregation sisters. This room had been her home, literally, for several years. She was on "isolation" precautions because of an infection that her labs never seemed to show cleared. She lived her life in the confinement of this room, with few exceptions. Sister had been a second-grade teacher all her life. I think that is why we connected so well. I love children, and many times feel most comfortable in the presence of little ones. I think our love of children connected us. We developed a child-like sense of banter between us. When I was young, I had originally intended to be a kindergarten teacher, so we hit it off famously. I don't know how anyone could not have loved her. I experienced pure joy every time I was with her. Just the thought of her brought a smile to my heart.

I started seeing Sister twice a week when she was admitted to hospice care. She was a little hard of hearing but always had a bright and broad smile and welcoming gesture when I arrived. I would pause at the "isolation" sign on her door, poke my head inside and ask if it was a good time to visit. Her consistent response was, "sure, come on in." I would don the isolation garb and kid her that I always had to dress up special for her. We quickly entered into a comfortable friendship which grew deeper as the days and months passed. With time and the consistency of my visits, she could count on me coming and seemed to delight in the time we spent together in the "cell" of her room. After my nursing assessment, we would sit and visit, spending time chatting or just being together.

Because of being confined to her room, she became essentially disconnected from the greater social aspect of life. She seemed to anticipate my visits, and I grew to really look forward to the time spent with her. When I would appear at her door and start donning the "isolation apparel," she would frequently comment, "Well, look who's here." I could spend as little as 30 minutes or as much as two hours with her, and when I would tell her it was nearing time for me to leave, she would always say, "Already, you just got here." She never seemed to comprehend the concept of time. But how could she being confined to this room as she had been? It was quite obvious she treasured the time, attention, and companionship during my visits.

Being of the same faith tradition, I would offer to sit with her as she participated in the daily Mass via telecast on her TV. After getting to know her and both of us feeling more comfortable with each other, we found light humor in our conversations that we both seemed to enjoy. As Mass was about to begin, I would jokingly comment that I could stay with her during Mass if she was OK with that, as I could certainly use the prayers. She always had a quick and cute response like "Don't I know it", or "Yes, you do," affirming our shared mischief and her true understanding of me.

If I happened to visit when it was close to mealtime, she was always generous to a fault and would offer to share with me whatever she had to eat. Her meal was always served on disposable dishes with plastic silverware due to the isolation precautions. She'd tell me I needed to eat and was more concerned about my eating than her own. This became difficult for me and I found myself telling lies to this innocent little nun as I would respond, "I just ate", or "I'm not hungry", or "I have my lunch waiting in the car". All lies. I was lying to this religious sister. I would burn in hell, but I couldn't possibly take food from her. As I declined her offer, she proceeded to consume every morsel of food set in front of her. I knew she would eat all of her meal, but her generous spirit was more important to her than her hunger or need for nourishment.

I remember the many attempts I made at trying to get her to go out of her room for a change of scenery with the appropriate protective attire on. One time in the autumn of the year, she finally gave in after my frequent requests and let me take her outside to pick leaves and nuts that had fallen from the trees. We did not stay for long; she just wasn't comfortable outside of that little haven of a room she occupied.

She taught me the most gracious way of enduring and tolerating limitations and unalterable confinements that happen in life in the way she accepted her isolation status. As her journey progressed and she became bed-bound and unable to communicate in her last days, I'd still appear at her door, donning the isolation garb, and in my mind, I could still hear her whispering to me, "Well, look who's here."

I had shared those treasured words she spoke to me with her fellow Sister who would be the eulogist at her funeral liturgy. During the funeral, the Sister giving the eulogy was reflecting on my little Sister's life and included the beauty of the Sister's comments when she shared, "As you enter the gates of Heaven, Sister, I can imagine God must have greeted you with the familiar "Well, look who's here." I won't be surprised but will be excited when my turn comes to journey beyond this world, and hopefully, I will hear Sister's familiar greeting, "Well, look who's here."

(Hospice nurse)

Oh, The Places You'll Go......In Your Conversations

Every person we care for gives us so much more than we feel we give to them. Mr. H. was a retired farmer who was admitted into our hospice program with a terminal stage of liver disease. He accepted the help of hospice which became a great benefit to him and also to his wife. Visits were scheduled, and with the supportive presence of hospice and the information and education provided, he was able to embrace the changes recommended, which eventually provided him with some quality of life. His acceptance and commitment to these changes were the reason for the improvement in his condition. We monitored his status closely, and with the ongoing support of his doctor, some changes to his Plan of Care, medication adjustments, and the support of his wife and hospice, he began to stabilize and started feeling better

He and his wife lived on the farm he had worked all his life. Our visits evolved into fun conversations along with efforts to get his symptoms managed. Being a farm girl myself, I could engage in and really enjoyed our conversations about many of the aspects of farm life that were important to him. We talked about many things related to farming. I often wondered just where our next conversation would lead us. We touched on many aspects of farming and farm life, and we even had a good and humorous conversation about outhouses. I would never have imagined my hospice work would have taken me to conversations about such things as outhouses. But there we were talking about those antiquated potty houses. You go where the path leads and where the patient wants to go. I have to say I really enjoyed those conversations, and I think he looked forward to them as well.

After many interesting conversations about farm life and the support, education, and instructions we offered to help manage his symptoms, we were able to have an occasional conversation about how he had come to this place in his life and how he was doing. I reflected to him how he had really taken charge of his life in a positive way by accepting the necessary changes needed and how it was really making a difference. I also told him he was the kind of person who could make a difference in many other lives through his example and commitment to the changes needed to better manage his body's decline from many years of hard living. With this improved sense of well-being, he would be a great spokesperson and role model for many. I think that conversation shed light on the potential for him to contribute something very worthwhile to others through the life he had lived. I also think it contributed to the improvement in his status and the fact that he was able to graduate from hospice, not once, but twice because he was doing so well. His ability to take control of his life with the help of hospice care truly made a difference.

I remember coming to the home one day while making a joint visit with the Social Worker, and he was in a dress shirt and looking so well. His appearance prompted me to ask if he was going somewhere special or did he have an appointment and did we need to hurry up with our visit. He said simply, "No." It was a nonverbal but very profound statement that acknowledged his gratitude for what we were able to bring to him at this challenging time in his life. He had dressed up just for us. The first time he was decertified from our program, we had a graduation celebration for him with balloons and a card of congratulations. He will always hold a special place in my heart as a man who gave his very best till the very end. I will always treasure those most unusual but memorable conversations we had. He was an inspiration in many ways. We had many moments that mattered to me, and hopefully, he was able to create some precious memories for his family in those last days of his life.

(Hospice nurse)

Beautiful Last Day

My elderly female patient had been in our program for some time and had been refusing a hospital bed which could have afforded her a more comfortable rest and allowed her a more relaxing position for visiting when she was awake. She continued to refuse the bed until we discovered the reason. She didn't want to be sleeping away from her husband of 60 years.

When we learned this, we were able to get her to accept the hospital bed with the plan that it be placed right next to the bed where her husband would sleep in their bedroom. She was able to sleep more comfortably at night and be close to him. The next day all the children and grandchildren were in the home visiting and were in and out of the room. She was much more comfortable in that hospital bed, and the visits were easier for her as well. Having been settled into a comfortable bed close to her husband and a full day of visits with her family, she was able to die content and peacefully that very night. One of the daughters told me, "It was the most beautiful last day ever, thanks to you."

(Hospice nurse)

If I Can Stop One Heart from Breaking

If I can stop one heart from breaking,

I shall not live in vain;

If I can ease one Life the Aching,

Or help one fainting Robin

Unto his nest again,

I shall not live in Vain.

By Emily Dickinson

Near You

The patient was an elderly gentleman whose condition was declining, and a hospital bed had been ordered and placed in the living room as there wasn't enough room for it in their bedroom. When I'd come to visit, I would find him comfortably lying in the hospital bed, but he reported he never slept in it at night. We had also provided an over-the-bed table next to the bed in the living room for him to put his water and other items on so they were close by. Everything seemed to be in order for his comfort.

One day as I was visiting, he happened to stretch out his hand from the hospital bed across the over-the-bed table, which prompted me to ask if he needed anything. He answered back, "No, I'm just reaching for my wife's hand. I just like holding her hand." With a little more conversation, I came to find out the main reason he wouldn't sleep in the hospital bed at night was that he wouldn't be able to lay next to her as he had in their bed for all their married years together. Being close to her was more important than his comfort, and he just needed her touch and for her to be close by.

(Hospice nurse)

I Can't Do This Much Longer

I had been seeing Gus for some time, and during my last visit with him, his daughter called me aside into a separate room and said, "I feel very uneasy about leaving Friday night and working Saturday." Gus hadn't been showing any of the signs or symptoms of imminently dying or any significant decline up to this point. We were only seeing slow but steady changes. I did talk to the daughter about the possibility of sudden death and to be aware of things the patient might say that could indicate that time was limited. The trajectory of decline is usually linear with a downward tilt, but there are times when something sudden and acute may happen, and death comes unexpectedly.

The patient had said good-bye to his hospice aide that day, almost like it was his final farewell. He also told his daughter the same day, "I can't do this much longer." In a somewhat unexpected manner, he died very suddenly that day with his daughter and caregiver by his side. He was so right when he shared that he could not "do this much longer."

(Social worker)

When the dying person speaks, we listen. It is not uncommon for patients to give clues or hints about the timing of their leave-taking. In his book Visions, Trips, and Crowded Rooms, David Kessler looks at three uniquely shared experiences that challenge our ability to explain and fully understand the mystery of our final days.

The first is "visions". As the dying lose sight of this world, some people appear to be looking into the world to come.

The second shared experience is getting ready for a "trip." The phenomenon of preparing oneself for a journey isn't new or unusual. In fact, during our loved one's last hours, they may often think of their impending death as a transition or journey. These trips may seem to us to be all about leaving, but for the dying, they may be more about arriving.

Finally, the third phenomenon is "crowded rooms." The dying often talk about seeing a room full of people... In truth, we never die alone. Just as loving hands greeted us when we were born, so will loving arms embrace us when we die.

In the tapestry of life and death, we may begin to see connections to the past and what we missed in life. While death may look like a loss to the living, the last hours of a dying person may be filled with fullness rather than emptiness......

(Excerpt from Visions, Trips, and Crowded Rooms by David Kessler)

It's Never Easy

The last eight weeks of my father's life were the best of times and the worst of times. We experienced so many emotions in that short amount of time. To say it was a rollercoaster ride would be an understatement. My father felt betrayed by his physician and his daughter. He was angry that this could be happening to him and went into complete denial to not face the reality of this current situation.

He continued to refuse the services and benefits of hospice, only relenting when I pleaded that the services would be a support to help me. I knew what hospice had to offer as I had worked at the hospice office for twelve years in a clerical/secretarial role. I knew very little about taking care of a dying person. It's one thing to hear about other families and to help them cope with their hard times. But when it hits home, it is quite another story.

Once he decided he could trust the staff, he began to really look forward to their visits. He enjoyed the chatting and joking around with them. His mood would lighten the moment they came into the room. This was a different man than the one who earlier had been so angry at the phone because he couldn't get through to his friends. He did not realize he was holding the TV remote in his hand at the time.

Through his illness, my father and I changed roles. I

became the one who had to be responsible. He smoked, and when it became apparent this was no longer safe as he was falling asleep mid-sentence, I started to hide the lighter. With his confusion, this worked for a while. But every time he left the room, he would come back with another lighter and would smile his defiant smile. As soon as he fell asleep, I would hide that one. We talked about an electric cigarette, but talking till you're blue in the face made no difference. It was No Go!! Being at my wit's end and fearing he might burn the house down, I engaged the help of the hospice nurse. With just one suggestion from her, yes, I said one, he decided he'd like to try the electric cigarette. He was actually happy with it and decided it was great because he could set it on his leg and not get burned. It's the small things in life that make the difference. These "small" things can carry great importance. They signify control, independence, and maintaining a life once treasured in small things and small ways.

The hospice ladies provided encouragement and support for changes that needed to be made, and they would take "the heat" with any of his resistance. No more driving, no more smoking, and using a cane for safety with walking. His resistance to some changes would never budge, like using a walker for safe walking, but they tried. And they let him have his say every step of the way and with every change. They assured his safety which was a great relief for the family. And they were there for me to talk to about what was going on, as my father never wanted to talk about dying. Hospice allowed me to be his daughter while also being his caregiver.

In those last couple of days, before he died, he had a regular routine at bedtime. He would say goodnight, get into bed and then holler down the hall to me, "I'm ready." I would go tuck him in, turn on his oxygen and kiss him goodnight.

The gift of hospice care gave us precious moments and gave me the strength to get through the pain of losing the person that I thought, as a child, would never leave, my dad.

(Hospice secretary)

A Mother's Love and Letting Go

Clara was a strong farm woman. She had been widowed young and had a big family to raise. She was strong to the core as she never remarried and continued to work the farm while raising her family. She had no other choice but to be strong, and she embraced her role of strength for her family with a fierceness that you wouldn't want to challenge. She did not know how to not be strong.

She had been in the hospice program for a time and was now getting close to dying as she had been unresponsive for several days. She had dedicated her life to her children, and they had now come from their homes and were all present in the home to care for her. This was a new and challenging twist to the roles the children played in her life. The hospice nurse was present and aware that each life has its own timing at the end. This strong lady had all her family present, but she continued to linger. Everyone had shared private time with her, and they realized it was time for her to let go and meet her reward in the next world. They started to wonder what it could be that she was waiting for. Sometimes the dying person needs permission to leave and to be reassured that the family and survivors will be okay when they are no longer here.

The hospice nurse suggested to these adult children, all boys, that they should take a break. The nurse would sit with their mom, so she wouldn't be alone, and she sent the boys off into the kitchen to make breakfast for the family.

They wondered if there was enough food but concluded that knowing their mom, she was always prepared, and yes, there was enough food. The boys were all together in the kitchen, had gathered the food items, and prepared breakfast, and everything was ready for them to sit down and eat. During this time, the hospice nurse remained at the bedside with Clara and told her that the kids were in the kitchen making breakfast for the family just the way she had taught them. She assured Clara that the boys were doing fine in their role of preparing food for everyone. It was just Clara and the nurse, alone in her bedroom. She sat with Clara and told her it was OK if she wanted to let go. The kids were all doing fine, and she need not hang on if she was ready to go.

The boys and their families had gathered around the kitchen table with the prepared breakfast set before them. They started the meal by praying for their mom, and as they were praying, the nurse appeared in the kitchen doorway. She came to let them know their mom had just died. Clara undoubtedly could hear them preparing their breakfast the way she had taught them, and when she heard them pray, she knew her work was complete.

This strong lady who had struggled to provide a good life and upbringing for these children all her life found it difficult to let go of her role in this family she cherished so much. Her main defined role in life was to provide for her children. Knowing that they would be OK and would have the help of hospice to get them through this difficult time after her death gave her the peace she needed to let go of her earthly hold on the role she held for so long.

(Hospice nurse)

A Mother's Love, Gift Wrapped

Ellen was in her 90s. She had lived a long life and worked hard. She was still very clear-minded as she would frequently share snippets of wisdom from her many years of life experience. Her son and daughter were devoted to her, as were her extended family. She had an endearing but straightforward way of imparting her wealth of wisdom. She now resided at a local nursing home, and her daughter's visits were regular and consistent. The daughter was very devoted to her mother. Ellen had been diagnosed with cancer and had considered the benefits of hospice care. She didn't feel she needed that, but with some coaxing and convincing, she agreed to "let them come in" because it would help her daughter. She was doing it for her daughter. There is no limit to a mother's love.

The benefit of hospice was especially important for the daughter, whose winter plans included a couple of months in Florida. Knowing how hard it was for the daughter to be away from her mom, the grandchildren surprised her at Christmas with the gift of airfare to come home during her time in Florida to visit Ellen. This would greatly ease the daughter's mind, and it was a gift to both mother and daughter. Midway through the time in Florida, the daughter made the trip home to be with her mom. Their time together was good, and mother and daughter were able to do some quality sharing about life and many other matters. They both verbalized how grateful they were for the time they had together. The daughter returned to Florida, but within a couple of weeks, the report was that Ellen was showing increasing signs of decline. Several weeks after the daughter returned to Florida, it became apparent to the daughter, through communication with the hospice nurse and nursing home staff, that Ellen was beginning to decline significantly.

Ellen had not felt well enough to go down to the dining room for meals for the past week. The daughter became quite concerned. She considered coming back home, but they were hosting family with them in Florida. She couldn't decide what to do. In helping her better understand her mom's condition, it was suggested to see what the following 24-48 hours might reveal to give a clearer picture of her mom's status.

On this particular Friday, Ellen's sister came to visit her at the nursing home. They had a nice visit reminiscing and being together. When the sister was leaving, she said she would be back to see Ellen the following week. Ellen answered, "If I'm here." This response from Ellen was very unsettling for her visiting sister and the daughter and seemed to offer an "alert warning".

On Saturday morning, the nurse reported that Ellen had gone down to the dining room for the first time in a week.

That seemed like a reassurance to the daughter, but it can be what can be referred to as "the calm before the storm," and often, family get their hopes up unrealistically. It becomes a wait-and-see game with close monitoring and surveillance during the ensuing 24-48 hours. Ellen revealed later in the day Saturday that it was a mistake to go to the dining room that morning. She remained in bed the rest of the day. The family was updated about the changes in her status, and the daughter decided to pack up and head home.

They left Florida for home early on Sunday morning with frequent contact with family and the nursing home staff. Ellen seemed to be deteriorating, and comfort meds were scheduled to help with her comfort and rest. She did happen to "perk up a bit" watching her beloved favorite baseball team, but only briefly. As Ellen's condition continued to deteriorate, her son and a granddaughter came to be with her at her bedside. Her daughter and son-in-law continued driving through the night in an effort to get home as quickly as possible. By Monday morning, Ellen had become unresponsive and was experiencing some breathing difficulties. The daughter from Florida continued on her way and was about seven hours away. With the rapid change in Ellen's status, the daughter was advised to call the nursing home and have them put the phone up to her mother's ear so she could talk to her. Even though the daughter had a wonderful visit just a few weeks prior, it was important for her to speak to her mom and let her know she was on her way and would be there soon. Early on Monday morning, the daughter called the nursing home, they placed the phone up to her mom's ear, and she was able to share some heartfelt sentiments and assure her mom she was on her way and would be there as quickly as possible. Ellen died five minutes after the daughter's call.

What a gift for a mother to complete her journey just moments after hearing her daughter's voice. Although the daughter was not able to be at the bedside at the moment of death, she was able to communicate with her mom at the most important moment of her mom's life. Knowing she no longer needed to race time and traffic to get to the bedside took away some of the anxiety and stress of riding hours in a car, wondering if she would get there in time. Those hours driving also gave her time to continue to talk to her mom and reminisce about the many gifts of wisdom she had imparted to her not only during her lifetime, but especially over the past several years when they were able to spend so much time together.

Another gift Ellen gave her family was that of timing. A granddaughter and her family were scheduled to go to Florida for vacation the following weekend. With the timing of Ellen's death, it seemed she orchestrated the timing to allow for everyone to be home for her funeral, but also able to "wrap up" the gift as the funeral was complete before the grandchildren were scheduled to go to Florida.

Many times we are able to look back and see how the events that have unfolded truly have happened the way they were supposed to. It would be hard to imagine any one of us could orchestrate better what is in God's hands. The hard part for those who journey with a loved one is to trust that it unfolds as it was meant to, just as a beautiful flower unfolds in its time. Just like the butterfly breaks free from its chrysalis at just the right time. Not too soon, and not too late. It really does happen the way it is supposed to.

(Hospice nurse)

"Death ends a life, but it does not end a relationship."

- Robert Woodruff Anderson

Looking Back

The Hospice Bereavement Coordinator makes contact with families following the death of their loved one. This often presents opportunities to hear about how the care provided by hospice staff has been a benefit to the patient and their families. Those making bereavement calls are privileged to help the surviving family member(s) in their grief during a time that feels like the darkest hour, and the realization hits them that their loved one is truly gone from this world. The conversations often center around and reflect on how much their loved one truly means to them.

While making a bereavement call to an elderly gentleman whose 93-year-old wife had recently died in our program, I was pleasantly surprised to hear a jovial, warm, and obviously smiling voice on the other end of the line. His voice resonated with a feeling of peace and joy that was obvious. When asked how things were going, he quickly replied, "Hon, I was blessed to have my beautiful wife for over 60 years. I'm sitting here in our apartment looking at all of the photos around the room of our life together." His hobby had been photography, so he captured many of their moments over the years on film. "I can see my beautiful bride's smiling face the day we were married, her beautiful smile after we had kids, our happiness together on our 50th Anniversary. I get to look at my angel every day. She was as beautiful the day she died as the day I met her."

He then asked if I were married. I said, "No, not yet, but I hope to be sometime soon." He answered back, "Well, I tell you what, I hope and pray that you are sitting here like I am one day, looking back on the life you shared with your husband, smiling, and just know you had the best possible life you could have with the one you loved. I am so lucky to have had a love like that, and I hope you are too."

Bereavement support is provided following the death of every hospice patient. During these moments when support is offered to help the person and family come to terms and deal with the loss of their loved one, we often become the privileged recipient of beautiful and heartfelt stories and sentiments that were precious and will be treasured forever by those survivors.

(Bereavement coordinator)

"The Dance"
By Garth Brooks

Looking back on the memory of
The dance we shared 'neath the stars above
For a moment all the world was right
How could I have known that you'd ever say goodbye

And now I'm glad I didn't know
The way it all would end the way it all would go
Our lives are better left to chance
I could have missed the pain
But I'd have had to miss the dance

Holding you I held everything
For a moment wasn't I a king
But if I'd only known how the king would fall
Hey who's to say you know I might have changed it all

And now I'm glad I didn't know
The way it all would end the way it all would go
Our lives are better left to chance
I could have missed the pain
But I'd have had to miss the dance

Yes my life is better left to chance
I could have missed the pain
But I'd have had to miss the dance

Written by: Tony Arata Lyrics Licensed & Provided by Lyric Find

43

Timing of Death

Death is a question of "when", not a question of "if".
Each of us will find our way to the end of our life at some
point in time. The death of a loved one is a very emotional
and difficult time for family and loved ones. Many times
family members convey their desire to be at the bedside at
the time of death. In their mind, family members often feel
that their presence at the bedside is necessary for their
loved one to know they care. However, it is the patient's
journey, and as uniquely as we enter the world, we also
uniquely leave this world according to what is best for each
individual. It is good to remember that death is very
personal. If the person has been quiet and reserved or had a
need for control in life, they may feel it best to be alone and
may find it hard to communicate this to family. There is no
crystal ball to determine the exact timing of death.
Experience with hospice patients has affirmed that death
occurs in the way, manner, and timing that it is supposed to
for the patient.

When someone feels they must be present at the time of
death, it has the potential to bring added anxiety and stress.
It is important when coming and going from the bedside to
say hello and goodbye to the patient. Letting them know
when you are leaving and when you expect to return or if
you are unable to return is important. Even when the person
is unresponsive, it honors them by letting them know what

is happening. When a family lives a distance away from the patient, messages of love can be provided to the patient using a phone or use computer interface technology. There are many options for communication and feeling present even when distance separates family from their loved one. It is always best to rely on what the person desires, if their wishes are known, as a guide for how to best be present to them.

Frequently, families push healthcare workers or hospice staff to give them specific information about "how much time" their loved one has left. It is often requested when a patient's condition changes in some way. It is difficult, if not impossible, to predict precisely the exact timing of a person's death. There are signs and symptoms, but again, there is no crystal ball, and sometimes even the best guess can be wrong. Death has a way of occurring in the manner and timing that it is supposed to. That may not be much help to families, but healthcare workers and hospice staff try to avoid giving specifics about when death will occur. Families and loved ones will tend to believe what medical staff says and will count on it as truth when it can give false hope. That is never what medical people want to do. However, there are certain indicators that help us to know when death isn't far off. An exception is when an acute event occurs that may not have been anticipated. When a change in a patient's status occurs, it can be more helpful to closely monitor the patient's status over the following hours or days. Monitoring the subsequent trajectory of decline over the next hours or days can provide greater insight into the course of the decline. But anything can happen at any time.

Family members who live away from their loved ones may ask staff, "should I come now" or how soon should I come? This, again, is a difficult question to answer. "Sooner is always better than later" is a good guide. Encouraging families to make their decisions based on what they might regret can be very helpful. No one wants to look back on the death of a loved one with any regrets. Using this as a guide and with the best information available about the patient's condition, most families can figure out what will work best for them. Each individual knows what their heart is telling them. If a family member comes and their loved one "hangs on", or seems to improve, there will be memories to treasure, and the visit will be a gift. If further decline or death occurs, there is comfort in having had time to share, even if the patient is not completely responsive. Patients are aware of who is present at their bedside even though they may not be able to communicate that. It is not uncommon to see some sort of response, facial expression, body movement, or other indication from the patient that they are aware when someone they may have been waiting for is present. But this may not always be apparent or obvious to those present. Giving a loved one every opportunity for comfort and honoring any known wishes is the best way to offer the dignity every human being deserves. It can be difficult to allow someone their own choices or way of doing things, but it is an everlasting gift that family can hold in their heart forever.

If a family member has visited and feels comfortable, they have said everything they need to say or shared the time they needed with their loved one or expressed all they need to, then leaving can be less traumatic if their loved one dies before their return. It is important to tell the patient when you are leaving and when you plan to return, if possible. If a family member is supposed to be present at the time of death, they will be there. Patients have been known to wait for a loved one to come before they take their last breath. This does not in any way mean that if the patient dies and you are not present at the time of death that they didn't want you there. Some people are very private, and there may be any number of reasons why someone might die without anyone at the bedside. It might be that the dying person does not want family members to be present to keep them from having the moment of death as their last memory. It might be they want the family to remember happier times together. The truth is we never really know how or why death occurs in the timing and manner it does. Being considerate, compassionate, understanding, and supportive to all family members without judgment at this time is the most beneficial way for everyone at this difficult time.

There may be times when a patient may need to be given permission to leave this world as they leave behind the ones they love. No one wants to leave their family unprepared to carry on when they are gone. They may need to be assured their loved ones will be OK. Oftentimes family members need the opportunity for quiet, private time with their loved one who is dying so they can share memories dear to them or convey some emotion they have had for the person. The time together might include words, touch, and music, or it might be as simple as presence alone. The patient somehow seems to sense the importance and preciousness of these moments.

No one should ever say anything but what is honest and truthful from their heart about what they feel for their loved one. It is not a time for platitudes but a time for heartfelt communication. The time might include tears, words, touch, or merely telling the loved one honestly that it may be a struggle to go on without them, but every effort will be made to continue on to the best of their ability. This can provide great comfort and assurance to the dying person. It lets them know they are loved, they will be missed, and their life has been full of meaning. It also lets them know they will not be abandoned in their final hours.

A lady who had raised ten children was in the intensive care unit of the hospital. She had loved every minute of life with her children, attending all their activities and never missing anything that was going on in their lives. While in the ICU, the children had all gathered around the bedside as they were informed that their beloved mother was most likely going to die. They had been taking turns at the hospital, so she was not going to be alone. It so happened that the children and her husband had stepped outside of her room to discuss the plan for who would stay at the hospital and what "shifts" each of them would take so their mother would never be alone. As they made plans and discussed the timing that would be best for each of them, they returned to the bedside to find that she had died while they were all away from her room. Sometimes our loved ones do not want us to remember their last breath but the whole of their life that has been so meaningful and filled with wonderful memories. It happens the way it is supposed to. It is just hard to accept that sometimes.

Doing It My Way

An elderly lady who was in the hospice program was nearing death but seemed to be having a hard time letting go. Her children were surrounding her, and they had been told about having individual time with their mom, sharing whatever heartfelt feelings they had for her or sharing thoughts and memories, or just having time to be with her. After an extended period of time, the family was getting tired and worn out as they continued to vigil at her bedside. They felt they had said all they wanted to say, had given her permission, and even told her she could let go. They assured her they would be OK. Anyone who needed to be there was present, and anyone that she needed to hear from had called. After some time, they asked the hospice nurse what could possibly be keeping her alive as she appeared to be so imminent.

Sometimes it seems that a parent might enjoy hearing the many stories, conversations, and memories shared among the family as they are sitting vigil with their loved one. As a mother, I would love to hear all those stories I may never have heard years earlier.

The hospice nurse engaged this family in talking about their mom, asking about her life and what she was like in life. What were her traits, characteristics, and what her personality was like. They all responded that she was always in control. She was in charge and pretty much "ran the show". She definitely had her own way of doing things and the family had all adapted to her ways. She wasn't to be told what to do. After some conversation, it became apparent that when the children told her it was OK to let go or even suggested that she let go, she, in her true characteristic way, had somehow made sure she would leave on her own terms and in her own time and not according to the families directives. When her family had decided to give her some space and left the bedside and no longer encouraged her to let go, she gently died in her own time. She had maintained control even through an unresponsive stage and did it her way. People don't change even in the last stages of their life. Many times in retrospect, we find the true character of a person continues throughout the last breath.

(Hospice nurse)

No, Before

Ron had been in our hospice program for about seven months. The hospice nurse and I had been making the frequently scheduled visits, and as happens, we had developed a good relationship with him. It was a Tuesday, and I had completed the bath and grooming care. His caregiver had told him that I'd be back the following Friday, to which he responded, "No, before." I asked him, "Should I call before I come?" and he said, "Yes."

Ron was right; he died Thursday afternoon.

When someone is close to the end of their life, sometimes they unknowingly give us information about the timing. When they speak, we listen. It's not that they have it figured out and have written the script, but there is an unrecognized intuition or insight that seems to give them the words to help us, and it's important that we listen.

(Hospic aide)

Ecclesiastes 3: 1-4

For everything, there is a season and a time for every purpose under heaven:

A time to be born and a time to die;

A time to plant and a time to pluck up what is planted;

A time to kill and a time to heal;

A time to break down and a time to build up;

A time to weep and a time to laugh;

A time to mourn and a time to dance;

It is not uncommon when a loved one is in hospice care for the family to ask the question, "how much longer?" or ask whether other family members from out of town or out of state should come. As hospice workers, we do not have the crystal ball to predict the exact timing of death. Some of the stories included here are evidence that the timing of death is between the person and their maker. Certainly, we can see evidence of decline and progress toward the end of life, but it can still be a surprise to families and even to hospice workers. When asked about coming to the bedside, it is hard to give specific timing. It is better to monitor closely any further change or decline over the following 24-48 hours. When asked if the family should make arrangements to come from a distance, the best answer is to "make decisions based upon what you would regret." If communication can happen via phone or electronic technology and family members are satisfied with that, it may be enough. If a family member feels they must be present for fear they will "miss" being there, they should come. The big decisions to be made must rely on an individual's choice, considering what might cause the most regret. In most hospice experiences, "sooner is always better than later."

Even if family feel they need to be at the bedside at the time of death, there are times when someone who vigils at the bedside may get up to take a break, go to the restroom or leave the room for any number of reasons, and the loved one dies while they are gone. It is deeply felt that the timing of death happens when it is right for the dying person. It can be difficult to help the family understand that it is their loved one's journey and it will happen the way it is supposed to for the individual. Many family and friends hang onto the belief that they "must" be at the bedside at the time of death. But this may not be what is best for the person. It might be the person does not want their last breath to be "a lasting memory" for their surviving loved ones. Another way the hospice care team can be helpful to survivors is by helping them understand and be comfortable with the process as it unfolds. I believe many of the stories shared here will affirm that truth. Such as…

Do We Go or Do We Stay

One elderly female patient, Agnes, was in the nursing home, and it was becoming apparent that she was progressing closer to death. She was getting close to imminent, basically unresponsive, but as often happens, it could be hours, days, or even longer. We tell families we do not have a crystal ball, and the timing is between the patient and their maker. Some people can go quickly, and others will linger. They keep us guessing, and we're often amazed at the timing. Three of this patient's daughters were becoming concerned as they had plans to go on a bus trip and were scheduled to leave the next week on Friday. Should they go, or should they cancel? They were overwhelmed by the decision and the changes they were seeing in their mom. Looking to hospice for guidance in making this decision, they were directed to "tell your mom" what their plans were and how they had this bus trip planned but did not know what to do. We told them we believed she would help them with the decision. We believe from experience that hearing is the last sense to leave, and people continue to hear even when they are not fully responsive. They did as they had been directed and shared with their mom the plans they had and the dilemma they faced, not wanting to leave her at this time.

As the week progressed, mom continued to decline.

Their anxiety was building as they did not want to leave her in this state. Families are often told when faced with difficult decisions to make their decisions according to their heart and what they will be able to live with. This helps clarify their priorities and what would make the most sense for their peace of mind. As we had anticipated and hoped, mom did help them with their decision, as she died on Thursday, the day before they were to leave on their trip. She died peacefully, and they had their answer.

Often we find the patient has an intuition when it comes to the timing of their death. Hospice has no control over the timing, but it can be important to help the family understand and be "OK" with the timing of the death. It is the patient's journey, and we are mere bystanders and fellow companions on their journey as they find their way home. Our role, and it is a hard one for most families, is to be open to accepting the timing and the manner in which their loved one's journey comes to a close. We frequently stand in wonderment in the midst of the mystery that unfolds before us and hopefully can help families come to terms with the unfolding of this most amazing conclusion to life. There is peace in knowing these important moments are not left to human probability.

(Hospice nurse)

I Don't Want another Birthday

I was assigned the care of this delightful lady in her 80s who lived in the town where I went to high school. One of her daughters was a classmate of mine. I hoped and prayed I would be able to serve them effectively and efficiently as this lovely lady was journeying through the last weeks of her life. She had enjoyed some quality time, her family had been in and out of the home throughout her illness, and she started to decline, progressing closer and closer to the end of life. Children who lived away from their hometown had all gathered in the home and were very supportive and encouraging of their mother as they provided hands-on caregiving.

It was getting closer to her birthday, and the children thought it would be nice to honor their mom with a little birthday celebration. It would be one last opportunity to pay tribute to their mom and demonstrate the love they had for her. They shared the idea of a birthday celebration with their mom, but she was pretty emphatic and repeatedly stated she did not want a party, she did not want a celebration, and she did not want another birthday. She continued to decline as the weeks rolled along, and as she declined, it appeared she would not be aware of the efforts of her children to celebrate her birthday. Her birthday was getting closer, coming on the following Thursday. She was kept comfortable, symptoms were managed, and she continued to change. Plans were still in place for a celebration of her birthday.

As mentioned earlier, we often stand in awe of the mystery unfolding before us, and with experience, we have come to believe death comes when it is supposed to. Not in our time, but in the timing that is right for the person. Interestingly enough, this lovely lady took her last breath at 11:45 pm Wednesday night. Just fifteen minutes before her birthday. She did not want a party or celebration, and she did not want another birthday. She got her wish. We are so often reminded there is a hand more powerful than any of ours in the events that happen in this life. We are just privileged to stand as witness to it. When we witness events like this, we are more and more assured that these things do really happen the way they are supposed to. No need to fret about timing; it will happen in the manner and way it is supposed to.

(Hospice nurse)

Our Anniversary Is Important

Mr. and Mrs. T. had celebrated many years of married life together and were still able to function and live independently in their own home. Mrs. T was in the last stages of lung disease, and they both had mounting medical issues wearing them down. They were determined to remain independent in their own home for as long as possible. Safety was becoming a concern as Mr. T. was not in the best health, but he was doing his best to care for his wife. The love between them was very apparent and nearly palpable as we witnessed the care he provided and the concern she shared about his mounting responsibilities for her. Grown children lived across the country and were unable to leave their jobs, family, and homes to help with caregiving. Oxygen equipment and respiratory treatments were provided in the home with frequent visits by both myself and our social worker, as we were both becoming very concerned for their safety. After much discussion and processing with them and their children, they relented and agreed to nursing home placement for Mrs. T. Arrangements were made for the transfer to the nursing home on the following Monday. Mrs. T was changing quickly.

Mr. T. was struggling with the impending loss of having his beloved wife at his side at home and her placement in the nursing home. They had never been apart from each other. They clung to each other for every breath of life. They would be celebrating their wedding anniversary the Friday following her nursing home placement. Mr. T was very straightforward in telling his wife how important celebrating their anniversary together was for him and that she could not die before their anniversary. The transfer to the nursing home was a huge physical challenge for Mrs. T.'s respiratory status, even though it was a few short blocks from their home. After the transfer and getting her settled in the nursing home, her status was getting worse, and she continued to decline throughout the week. Changes were made to her Plan of Care in hopes of keeping her alive and comfortable to fulfill her husband's wishes. We were all worried she would not survive to celebrate their anniversary. But we have no control over the timing of life or death.

Mr. T spent every waking moment at her bedside at the nursing home, and they were able to be together all day Friday, the day of their anniversary. Then shortly after midnight Friday night, in the early morning moments of Saturday, Mrs. T. asked the nurse attending her what time it was. The nurse told her it was 12:20 am. Then she asked what day it was, and the nurse told her it was Saturday. Being comforted that it was no longer Friday, their anniversary, Mrs. T. was able to drift peacefully into sleep and died a half hour later. Another moment that mattered as we witnessed the hand of a greater power at work.

They were able to "celebrate" their anniversary on Friday as Mr. T had hoped. We all breathed a sigh of relief and offered a prayer of thanks to God.

(Hospice nurse)

What we have once enjoyed, we can never lose. All that we love deeply becomes a part of us.

- Helen Keller

But I Wasn't There

A co-worker had been on vacation, and I was following her patient, Doc, in her absence. Doc and his family had become very attached to their hospice nurse. They allowed me to visit, but it was obvious they missed their "special" nurse. The first day I saw him, he was quite compromised. He could barely walk from the bathroom to the hospital bed, which had been set up in their three-seasons room. His wife was concerned about this decline and requested spiritual support from their faith community. The parish visitor, who was a religious sister, was scheduled to come the following day, but the wife thought it would be better if she could come that same day. A quick call was made to the parish with the request for a visit that same day if possible. The nun was accommodating and able to make the visit within the next couple of hours.

I made a call into the home the following day to check and make sure the wife was comfortable with giving the medication doses that were recommended. She stated he was declining, but with further conversation, it sounded like he was no different than he had been the day before. I had been unaware of the wife's beginning dementia and had taken her assessment of her husband as truth. He was changing but did not look to be imminent, and a visit was offered but declined until the following day. Unknown to us, she had called family, and three of the four sons arrived at the home.

A daughter who lived a short distance away was also on her way. Doc declined quite quickly throughout the day, and the daughter was just arriving at the home. Doc died within five minutes of the daughter's arrival. She was distraught and devastated that she had not been there earlier to spend more time with her dad. Sometimes, there is never enough time. Even though she only had five minutes with her dad before he died, he did wait for her to get there before he was able to leave peacefully. The hospice was called and notified of the death, and the hospice nurse arrived quickly. Support and conversation were offered in an attempt to help the daughter understand the timing of her father's death as beautiful. He had waited for her to arrive, but it just didn't seem like enough time to her.

In time, hopefully, the daughter will be able to appreciate that her father waited for her to arrive before he died, even if it was only five minutes.

(Hospice nurse)

No

Mr. B. had been admitted to hospice and had gotten comfortable with the nurse, social worker, and all the services provided to keep him comfortable and help him on his journey. Time was passing, and as happens occasionally with the close surveillance, monitoring, and adjustments to his plan of care, his condition was beginning to stabilize. It was determined he might need to be decertified as he might no longer qualify for hospice care and services. He was informed of this potential change in his care arrangements.

He had become accustomed to the services and staff and was not happy about the impending decertification. He was assured that ongoing care planning was in place and he would not be abandoned in the care provided following his discharge from hospice. He would receive care and monitoring through his personal physician's office, and there would be no breach in the quality of care he would receive. He understood but continued to be distressed at this impending change.

Surprising to everyone, he died suddenly prior to his decertification date. He really did not want to lose the services and staff support he had become accustomed to and appreciative of. It would seem there is a sense of control even when there appears there is no control.

(Hospice social worker)

Bucket Lists and Goals

End-of-life wishes can be very important to a person. The importance of Advance Directives and having a conversation about those wishes with the person or persons who will be speaking on behalf of the dying when they are no longer able to speak for themselves cannot be overstated. It is important for everyone to be clear about any particular wishes about what they do and don't want to be known so they can be honored and respected as they find their way home in the last days of life. Advance Directives are mainly about the technical, medical interventions or treatments at the end of life. Wishes can also be about something as simple but as important as presence, touch, talking, music, or any host of things that would bring comfort to the person in their last days. It helps loved ones who want to support them to know any specific wishes they might have. It is a way to honor and respect any final wishes. It is a final gift that is worth giving.

When a person is admitted to hospice early in the course of their final journey, something that can be addressed is the topic of any goals or items that might remain on their bucket list. It is a time to review priorities that might still exist for them. There may be events or occasions they might be looking forward to. It might be addressing simple things like how someone might want to be treated or what measures might be comforting to them during this last phase of life. It allows the person to identify people they might want to be part of their care team. Would they benefit from spiritual support or reconnecting with previous friendships or relationships? There might be specific care actions that would bring comfort or knowing those things that might bring more stress. Some people like touch, and some do not. It allows the person to look more closely at the things that would provide comfort and quality to their days and also identify anything that might cause distress. There might be individuals they want to be part of their care team and others they might prefer not to be involved. It is not a time of judgment but one of defining what will provide the most comfort and peace to their days. It offers an opportunity to personalize the care and treatment during the final phase of life. Having some control over little things can become very important when control of bigger things like the progression of the illness or disease is out of their hands.

There are multiple options available to help someone work through these aspects of care. One that is available is the "GO WISH" game. It is a card game and can be purchased, or there is an online version.

http://www.gowish.org/article.php/faqs

Another option to identify the specifics of care beyond the medical and technical treatments or interventions is the

Five Wishes approach to Advance Care Planning.

https://fivewishes.org

https://agingwithdignity.org

I Don't Want Anyone "Hovering" Over Me

Sister M. was a very independent and self-proclaimed stubborn individual. So when she got the diagnosis of cancer, it was a very challenging time for her. Not wanting to give up any independence and being very private, she was not very forthcoming with her diagnosis and change in her health status with her fellow congregation sisters. As her disease progressed, she even declined the offer to move to the infirmary of her congregation. She had been the "oldest" sibling in her family of origin and was accustomed to taking charge and not being told what to do. As her health deteriorated and it became apparent she would not be able to care for herself, she reluctantly agreed to move to the nursing care area of her congregation, but not without some conditions.

It can be customary, when living in a religious congregation with other nuns, that when someone is nearing the end of life, the sisters take turns sitting vigil with their dying sister, so no one dies alone. The time of vigil may include prayers for the safe passing of the dying person or just a quiet presence. Sister M. did not want to tell her biological family of her decline as she was adamant she did not want them "hovering" over her or standing around and "talking about her" as she was living the last days of her life. With changes to her health happening more quickly, she finally did agree to notify her siblings and allowed them to come to the congregation infirmary and into her room for short visits. But the family was not allowed to gather outside the door of her room and talk about her status. They respected her wishes for them to stay away most of the time. She had shared with me early on when she admitted that she did not want her fellow sisters in the congregation sitting vigil and praying over her when she was in her last days and hours. Having this information from Sister allowed us to help the family and her congregation sisters understand her wishes and ensure that her final wishes were honored. It is important, whenever possible, to honor the wishes of the dying person, even when it seems to go against normal instincts or customs. Hospice workers become essential in helping make those wishes happen and helping the survivors understand the gift of honoring those wishes.

Sister M's independence was something she was very protective of, and she just didn't want anyone "hovering over her" as she was breathing her last. A very simple but important gift to her was assuring her that her wish would be honored.

We don't always understand the timing of death, and those who are experiencing the death of a loved one will often question how or why it happened differently than the way they had anticipated and hoped it would. Helping families understand it is the patient's journey and that we have no control over the timing is part of the hospice support provided. Included in walking with the family of a loved one who is on the last leg of their journey here on earth is also to support the family in helping them understand it may not happen according to anyone's expectations other than that of the dying person. Helping the survivors understand and be OK with the process as it unfolds can be challenging but is part of the care and support that comes with hospice. As mentioned, it is a process that is between the patient and their maker. It can be difficult to make sense of something that seems senseless. It is in the hands of a power greater than any human, and we are mere companions on the journey

(Hospice nurse)

Keep Flying High

TM had always lived her life the way she wanted, and even with her terminal diagnosis, she planned to continue to do things her way. (People really don't change just because they have received a life-limiting diagnosis).

Prior to TM's admission to hospice care, she spent most of her days in bed, writhing in pain. Leaving the house was not an option due to her unmanaged pain. Her doctor had mentioned hospice care to her when they discovered she was allergic to the chemotherapy treatments. She initially resisted the hospice referral, but as the pain increased and became intolerable, she relented and asked her brother to "just call hospice".

The same day her brother made the call to hospice, she was admitted to the program. The care team immediately began working on managing her pain. With frequent monitoring of her comfort and adjustments to her Plan of Care, her pain lessened and became tolerable. She resolved to live in the moment and not worry about tomorrow. She was amazed and relieved that she was not thinking about pain every moment of the day. She was able to go on living her life in spite of her prognosis. When her hospice care team asked about any specific wishes or goals she might have, she was full of ideas. One of those wishes was to ride in a hot air balloon. If there is any opportunity to make something memorable happen for a patient, every attempt is made to accomplish what might seem to be impossible. With some changes to her plan of care and improvement in TM's symptoms and her pain better managed, the planning began. Her hospice nurse received the okay from her doctor for the ride, and her social worker began putting things in motion. A local businessperson donated the balloon ride for TM and her hospice SW.

Everything was set, the day arrived, and the balloon and basket were prepared. The hot air balloon pilot, TM, and the Social Worker climbed into the basket. It gently lifted off the ground and started to soar higher and higher. They just trusted it to go wherever the wind would blow. As they lifted higher and higher, the guide was able to point out areas of interest in the countryside over which they were floating. TM said, "I was so excited just getting in the basket." The ride turned out to be one of the highlights of her life, and the SW shared the same sentiment. After a glorious ride high above the treetops, the pilot maneuvered a gentle landing of the basket. When they climbed out of the balloon basket, there was champagne and chocolates waiting to welcome them back to earth.

Having experienced a cherished goal and realizing and appreciating the support and care of her hospice team, TM compared her balloon ride to her experience with hospice. She was not worried and felt so comfortable sailing aloft with the pilot guide offering guidance about what to expect.

Hospice made it possible for her to complete one of her dreams. She shared that without hospice coming into her life and managing her pain, she would not have had the opportunity to accomplish what at one time had seemed to be an impossible dream. She felt confident her hospice care team would also guide her on her journey during this final phase of her life, giving her the support and direction she needed to maintain control over her life and to live life to the fullest no matter how limited her number of days might be or where it would lead. She regained a sense of trust and some control which was important to her.

With hope in her heart, she then shared that her next goal might be to explore even greater horizons, maybe skydiving or parasailing. She was overjoyed to have been able to accomplish this one impossible dream. Lesson to be learned: never stop hoping, wishing, or dreaming.

(Hospice social worker)

With the greater community experiencing and realizing the benefit and support of hospice care, it is not uncommon for people to want to become involved and invest in helping fulfill a wish for someone on their final journey in life. In the last story, one community business graciously provided the balloon ride. There are many times when a community-minded individual or business is willing to offer their support to help accomplish a goal for a patient, no matter whether the goal is big or small. Hospice has helped people go fishing one last time, or go to the casino, get a tattoo, or visit a home or farm that has been an essential part of their life story. Whatever is on their bucket list, it is important to help make those last wishes a reality if at all possible. It is better to get hospice involved sooner than later as the possibilities for goals and dreams to be achieved are much better when there is more time available. We hear of many requests, and occasionally they are about enjoying a special food one last time.

Lobster Please

Our hospice nurse had been seeing this little religious sister who had been in our program for some time. She decided to ask her if there was anything special she might need or like. This little nun shared that she especially enjoyed a specific type of seafood, lobster, and that would be her wish for a good last meal if it could ever be possible. Sometimes a joy or pleasure can be as simple as a taste of a favorite food. Our town doesn't consistently have freshwater fish readily available, but undaunted by this fact, the nurse made phone call after phone call, looking for a restaurant that might be able to provide this special request. Having located a restaurant that had lobster, the nurse ordered the meal. When she presented at the restaurant to pick up the food, she had her "hospice" name tag visible. The restaurant owner noticed the hospice name tag and asked if the meal was for the nurse or for a patient. She explained the story of the nun and her wish for this last-time favorite meal that she'd like to enjoy.

Upon hearing the story, the restaurant owner offered the seafood meal free of charge. He wanted to help offer this religious sister the enjoyment of a delicacy she had hoped for. It was his way of offering support for the efforts of our local hometown hospice to provide care in the community. The nurse thanked him greatly and said how grateful we were that the restaurant had it available.

We often find that our community goes above and beyond in so many ways to help support our mission of caring for those who are facing a life-limiting illness or disease. We are blessed to live in a community that understands the importance of local hospice care and is always willing to step up to help in whatever way they are able to make the last leg of life's journey easier for someone. We cannot overstate the importance of community support, and we are forever grateful for every way in which our community offers its support to help us accomplish our mission of serving the terminally ill. They need to know their efforts, however small or insignificant they may seem, do make a huge difference in someone's life. We are forever grateful to all of them. There are many generous people in this world, and working in hospice provides an opportunity to meet many of them.

(Hospice nurse)

There is within each of us a potential for goodness beyond our imagining, for giving which seeks no reward, for listening without judging, for loving unconditionally.

Elisabeth Kubler Ross

The Need for Speed

Bets was in her 60s and had come to live in the nursing home due to the degenerative nature of her hereditary neuromuscular disease.

She was astute in her thinking and fully engaged in life despite the functional limitations of her disease. As is common in hospice, when we admit someone to the program, we discussed any potential goals or wishes she might like to accomplish in the days and weeks ahead. We are always happy when someone is admitted early to the hospice program so we can identify any bucket list items that might be meaningful to them. Bets surprised me when she mentioned she thought a motorcycle ride would be fun.

After getting to know her and having built trust with her, on one of my visits, she asked, "what about this motorcycle ride?" I responded, "I always believe sooner is better than later." She did not immediately respond to my comment but must have taken my words to heart. The next day her son showed up at the nursing home with his motorcycle and a dew rag for mom. Staff brought her out in a wheelchair, and we lifted her onto the motorcycle and seated her behind her son, dew rag in place. A gait belt was used to secure her torso to his body for stability. Her hands were raised and placed over her son's shoulders. They took off, and we prayed.

He took her out onto the local county roads that had been so familiar to her, and as they were traveling the winding scenic roads, she leaned forward and said into his ear, "Faster!" Here was a lady who struggled to move one foot ahead of the other as she was trying to make her way down the halls at the nursing home, and she was asking for the thrill of going "faster". They returned back to the nursing home from the ride, she was still in place behind him, and the unmistakable joy she felt was evident on her face. She was helped off the motorcycle and into the wheelchair. Staff wheeled her back to her room and were concerned about her comfort, asking if she were sore, hurting, or in any way distressed or uncomfortable. Everyone's assumption was that the ride would have been very difficult for her. With a broad smile that reflected her exhilaration, she replied, "I am high on life." She returned to her room, and her euphoric spirit filled the rest of her day. She would spend some time thinking of other exciting adventures she might like to experience.

What a surprise it was for all of us when we received a call the following morning from the nursing home staff telling us that Bets had died. Sometimes an acute and unexpected event surprises us, and we are bewildered at the abrupt change in someone's status. Most of the time, we are able to see a linear trajectory of decline and change, but once in a while, we stand in awe and amazement at how events unfold differently from what was expected. For Bets, everyone agreed that she was more than thrilled to have had one last experience of speed when her physical status had, for so long, restricted her from this exhilarating pleasure. I can only imagine the broad smile that graced her expression as she rode off into the next world in a speedy way.

(Hospice nurse)

Basketball or Bust

Stella and her husband were avid basketball fans. They had season tickets for in-state university basketball games for many years and would treat one grandchild at a time to a game. Stella had received a diagnosis of cancer and was experiencing some significant decline in her functional status, dropping BP, ascites, etc. She had faced many challenges in her life and found solace in the sport of basketball. She was tall and stick thin and was developing increasing ascites with an ever-enlarging abdomen.

One of the daughters who had been to a recent university basketball game mentioned to the media present at the game that they do so much for so many youth, what about a lifelong supporter who was facing death? That prompted the athletic department representative at the university to offer to have the patient "meet the players" if she were able to get to a game.

The family felt it important to get her to one more basketball game, but the prospect was looking bleak with her rapid disease progression and relentless ascites. Arrangements were made to drain the fluid for comfort, but due to the scheduling of the procedure interfering with the proposed plans to attend the basketball game, the procedure was canceled to be rescheduled. Stella's symptoms were managed as well as possible with every effort made to get her comfortable and get her to that game. The procedure was rescheduled at a time that did not conflict with the game and with instructions for comfort for the family who would go with her. She was able to make the trip to the game with much family support. Everyone knew how much this meant to her. She was able to meet and shake the hand of each of the players, and she received a special autographed "game ball" from them as well.

Getting to one more game of the sport she loved so much, and the opportunity to meet the players and receive an autographed game ball was better medicine than could be offered by treatment or pills. It was highlighted in the news, and when she returned with the game ball, sharing in her excitement, I commented how wonderful that was. She then mischievously offered to let me "touch" the game ball for $10. She still had her spirit.

The time from her diagnosis to death was only a matter of weeks. She was able to experience some memorable moments due to her family's efforts and adjustments to proposed procedures for her comfort. Moments the family will treasure always. She received a gift beyond measure with that trip and making this happen for her and her family lifted them and their spirits during some very difficult days. She had accomplished an impossible goal that was very significant and memorable to her and her family.

At her funeral, the game ball was displayed (in a

protective case), and a representative of the university even came to the service. These were moments that mattered more than words can express and will live on for her family as they remember this spirited lady. Having the encouragement and support of hospice made this goal for Stella and her family possible at a time when it all seemed impossible.

(Hospice nurse)

Working in hospice teaches us it isn't the grand and ambitious things we do that make the difference in life. More often, it's what happens in the quiet, muted, and seemingly insignificant moments that make the most difference. Hospice attempts to help patients get the most out of every day of life that is available, even in the most hushed moments of everyday life. Making the seemingly impossible become possible for someone whose control over the events of their life has been taken from them is more important than words can describe. It fills our hearts with satisfaction that cannot be appreciated in the words of a job description. Those who give are also those who receive. This is God's work. It's the most beautiful and best.

Go With Gusto

Warren's health was a long road with many medical problems. He was in his 90s and had endured years of compromised health from heart failure, COPD, and dementia. He resided at the nursing home as he needed more care than could be provided at home. His loving wife came daily to visit. Most of the family lived away from their hometown, and as with most families, it was hard to get everyone together. But with dad's failing health, they decided on a weekend get-together when everyone could make it, and a family celebration was planned.

Saturday was the day. Everyone gathered at the nursing home with pizza, beer, and wings. Dad participated with enthusiasm, even consuming eight wings which was twice the amount he would normally eat, and he was even able to enjoy a beer. The party lasted all afternoon. It was a grand celebration. Mom and Dad had their family together. What could be better?

The following day, on Sunday, with everyone home and close by, the party continued at a son's home. They had steaks and those locally famous cheesy potatoes everyone loved and even more beer. Warren came from the nursing home, and everyone was there, children, grandchildren, and great-grandchildren. The party atmosphere continued, and everyone commented on how much dad was enjoying himself. He even ate two steaks. Could life be any better than the fun, food, and festivities that hold a family close at hand when they've been apart for so long? Dad returned to the nursing home with a content heart.

The following morning dad awoke with a major heart attack. The ambulance was called, and he was transported to the hospital. He was in his last hours. Family and everyone gathered with mom at his bedside. Everyone was very sad, but in the midst of their sadness, they were able to cherish the great weekend they had just spent together celebrating. Even the staff and his doctor commented, "What a perfect way to spend your last days".

Warren found a way to go out with gusto. Everyone will remember the beauty of those days and moments preceding Warren's death and the gift of being together, having fun, enjoying favorite foods, and watching dad enjoy himself. Everyone was able to be together to support mom and each other as dad got his last "kick" during his final days as he sprinted to the finish line on the last leg of his final race in life. You can't orchestrate something this meaningful or beautiful. It's just a marvel and a mystery to be witness to it.

(Son of patient and hospice nurse)

Massage on the Move

Sylvia was in her 80s and had been a prominent lady of influence in her community for most of her life. It was hard for the family to see her at the nursing home where she resided due to her progressing Alzheimer's disease. She was essentially non-verbal, had a restlessness to her, and was highly anxious. She could be seen pedaling her feet forward as she independently paced the halls in her wheelchair. She would consistently avoid eye contact.

The massage therapist was invited to start seeing Sylvia in hopes the therapy might help calm some of her anxious restlessness. Sylvia would occasionally spend time during the day napping on her bed, but only for short periods of time. When she was up, she was in her wheelchair, pedaling toward some unknown destination with a determination that wasn't to be interrupted or controlled. She was constantly on the move. The massage therapist soon became aware she was not going to be of any help if she expected Sylvia to lay in bed or sit still for her massage therapy sessions. With her own determination and persistence, the massage therapist found a way to accommodate Sylvia. She would follow her in the wheelchair wherever she went giving whatever adapted form of massage she could accomplish with this patient on the move. With each session, Sylvia did seem to become more relaxed as she and the massage therapist strolled the halls of the nursing home.

Finding whatever is needed to adapt services to the specific needs of the patient is essential to providing quality care and also allowing the patient to be who they are. We are not there to change them, but we can be challenged to be quite creative in providing the services offered as we honor the individuals we serve. In this case, the massage therapist was quite literally challenged to "follow her lead". With persistence and creativity, she was able to provide some measure of comfort and also decrease some of the anxious behavior experienced by the patient because of this disease.

(Massage therapist)

The Red Hat Lady

Her name was Dottie. I was fortunate to spend time with her during her last year. She was 85. I would never say old because she was anything but old. Dottie was a one-of-a-kind person. Dottie had spunk, dressed fashionably, and loved a little sparkle and the color purple. She wore her hair short and spiked. Dottie freely gave out hugs that totally engulfed you. She had a smile that would light up a room and a fierce love for her family that would rival any Mother Bear.

Dottie lived halfway down Oak Street, a street that, for the most part, was quiet, except for the times when the nearby school was starting or letting out for the day. Dottie's house had a big, inviting front porch that was shaded under large, graceful trees. You felt welcomed before the door opened. This was the house in which Dottie and her husband had raised their family of eight children. Her door was always open to friends and family that came and went throughout the years, and you felt comfortable in Dottie's presence. If you entered as a stranger, you left as a friend.

Time always went fast when you were with Dottie. She told stories of the early years when her children were small, welcoming the first snow and playing in the yard. Her backyard was a gathering place for neighborhood children, but Dottie didn't mind. She said that way she always knew where her own children were. Dottie loved all little children. Even as her health started failing, she gave them all hugs and some attention and never missed giving compliments about their new shoes or hair ribbons. She made them feel special.

Summertime meant swimming or making boats for competitive races on the Mississippi. Her eyes filled with tears as she remembered her husband's final race and the effort her children made so their dad could participate. Her last summer, even with Dottie's failing health, her children again would have it no other way than to have Dottie included in the fun. Always the fashionable one, Dottie wore a red, wide-brimmed hat as she sat there on the dock in the summer sun, enjoying every moment of the day. The day's activities and excitement made her thoroughly exhausted. Dottie said the day brought her so much joy that it was worth every bit of the exhaustion she felt. The next day, a large box was sitting on the table when I arrived at Dottie's house. She said it was a gift for me. To my surprise, it was her red wide-brimmed hat! She said she wanted me to have it and that I should wear it "anytime you want to add a little flair."

Dottie had a beautiful singing voice. She reminisced about singing Silent Night on Christmas Eve from high in the church balcony. Looking down, she saw her husband with all of their children sitting in a row near the front of the church. She said, "I was so proud of them." I can only imagine how beautifully she sang that song. I'm sure she sounded just like an angel. A couple of months before Dottie died, I heard her beautiful singing voice. This time it was a lullaby to her 16th great grand baby. Watching her hold that tiny baby and sing a lullaby to him was priceless. One day Dottie told me, "I'll have to sing to my next great grand baby when I meet him in heaven. I don't think he'll get here before I have to leave."

As her health continued to decline, Dottie needed more help and was fortunate as her family provided all she needed through those difficult times. She was so proud of her children. She told me, "I'm amazed that no matter what I ask, no one ever lets me down!" Their help was all done with love and an added sense of humor. Sometimes this showed up as two-step dancing, leg strengthening, neon shoes, tuna-noodle casserole (no peas), morning Mass, nightly monitoring, medications, meals, bathing, dressing, shopping, and more, but most importantly, just being with her. Everything was performed with love for a mother that taught them by example.

I loved Dottie. Although I knew Dottie was coming to the end of her journey on this earth, I was still not prepared when I heard that she had died. "Thirty minutes ago, very peacefully," her daughter said. I sat quietly, thinking of this great lady and of the many things I learned from her. Family is of the utmost importance, and there is unconditional love. Treat everyone with kindness. Make other people feel like they are most important. Stay stylish. Don't be afraid to add a little sparkle. Spike your hair and wear a red wide-brimmed hat, even if you're not in the sun.

I was still thinking of Dottie and the sadness her family must be experiencing when suddenly, my eye was drawn to an angel that sat high on a shelf in the corner of my living room. She was glowing like a spotlight was shining directly on her! Nothing else in the room was lit up except that angel. My thoughts immediately turned to Dottie. I know Dottie was sending me a message, letting me know her journey on earth was finished, and now she was on her way to heaven to be the newest angel.

My thoughts often return to Dottie, and I smile as I remember her. Sometimes I imagine a beautiful angel singing softly as she prepares a tiny baby boy to be delivered to earth...Shhhh...What's that I hear??? Could it be??? "Bye baby bunting, daddy's gone a hunting...

(Hospice aide)

So Pretty

The humidity of a Midwest summer afternoon could not hamper the excitement of the 4th of July fireworks for Maryann. People were coming into town early to get the best spot for viewing the fireworks over the river. I got caught in traffic on my way to see Maryann, my last patient for the day. Finally, I reached Maryann's house and found a parking spot fairly close. I realized how intense the afternoon heat had become as I walked up to the door. Many of Maryann's family had gathered in the small living room, the small window air conditioner working hard to fight the intensity of the July heat. Some were sleeping, kids were drawing pictures, and moms were entertaining babies. It was a small room, but there was enough room for everyone. They had planned a cookout to be followed by the fireworks from the best seat in the town: grandma's front porch.

Maryann's room was next to the living room. Seven years earlier, she had been diagnosed with breast cancer at the age of 38. Following surgery and extensive chemotherapy and radiation, she was declared cancer free. She had won the battle. It had been devastating to get the news that her cancer had returned, and this time it was in her bones, liver, and lungs. That's when Maryann decided to enter the hospice program. She desired to be pain-free and comfortable in her own home, enjoying quality time with her family. I had the privilege of being Maryann's hospice aide.

That July day, she sat in her recliner in her room with the air conditioner and a fan helping to move the air. It seemed to help her breathing. She was weaker today due to the disease progression, but she was determined to attend this family party. I think she knew this would be the last family function she would be able to attend. I helped her bathe, washed and styled her hair, and got her dressed. We chatted as we worked, and Maryann told me about the members of her family who were in the small living room. She explained that her illness had been very hard on her entire family, especially her husband. She told me how he worked hard to make ends meet, sometimes picking up extra hours. I could see her eyes well up with tears as she spoke.

We worked slowly, allowing Maryann to rest often. The July heat was gaining strength, and I had to stop and wipe sweat from my forehead. Maryann chose to wear a sleeveless, full-length burgundy dress with a beautiful tapestry bodice. It was lovely, but I was surprised at her choice of clothes, and it reminded her of the heat of the afternoon. "I want to wear the jacket, too," she said. She selected earrings and a necklace and dabbed perfume behind each ear. She sat down in her recliner to catch her breath. She looked up at me and smiled. "The last time I wore this dress, I wore four-inch heels. My husband and I went out for dinner and then went dancing. We had the time of our lives."

Suddenly it all made sense to me. I could see another side of her, a beautiful lady, all dressed up, happy and healthy, and unaffected by cancer. Maryann stood up, turned, and looked at her reflection in the mirror. She smiled and said, "I feel so pretty."

Maryann died five days after the 4th of July party. I find great comfort in knowing that every 4th of July, she looks down from heaven to see a spectacular fireworks display. She still has the best seat in town from her new view, and they must look "so pretty."

(Hospice aide)

Selling the Salesman

Paul was an elderly gentleman who had been in sales all his life. He was good, and as they say, he could have sold snow to an Eskimo. Paul's health had been deteriorating, and he wasn't interested in giving up or giving in. He was made aware of the benefits of hospice care but continued to decline the offer of services, and it seemed there was no way to convince him of the benefits. The salesman in him was firm. He continued to progress, and his health condition was getting increasingly worse as time went on. He was becoming more compromised and, in a "weak moment," was agreeable to accepting the services of hospice care.

Hospice had started seeing Paul, and both the hospice nurse and the hospice aide happened to be male. He started to look forward to their visits, and as time went on, he was able to freely admit that he was very glad he had decided to enter hospice. The salesman had been sold. And he was very pleased as he realized the many ways that hospice was able to help him and provide the best quality to the days he had left.

(Hospice nurse and Hospice aide)

When words fail, Music speaks

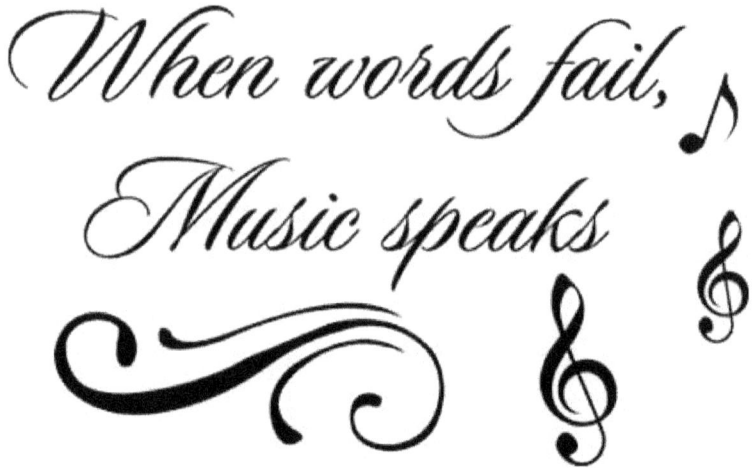

Music is one of the great mediums that connects human beings. Music evokes emotions and helps us express feelings we may have trouble verbalizing. It can help alleviate pain and manage or reduce stress. It can enhance memory and take us to a place we long for from times past. It can tell a story that we resonate with. It can transport us to a time and place we may long for. It can promote well-being and enhance communication. It can help make exercising easier, and it can lift us up and help us get through difficult times. In writing this book, I realized that music is a big part of life. The following lyrics from a favorite song by Steve Wariner seem to put the journey of life in perspective.

"Life's Highway"
By Steve Wariner

Sun is up, time's at hand

There's a stir across the land

And so begins another day

On life's highway

On city streets down country roads

Like a stream, the people flow

There's bread to win and tolls to pay

On life's highway

There is hope with every turn

A bridge to build, a bridge to burn

Here's hoping you never go astray

On life's highway

We are young, then we're old

Passing through, then passing on

Like the roses bloom and fade

On life's highway

Step by step, round, and round

Never knowing where we're bound

From the cradle to the grave

On life's highway

There is hope with every turn

A bridge to build, a bridge to burn

Here's hoping you never go astray

On life's highway

Sun is up, time's at hand

There's a stir across the land

And so begins another day

On life's highway

Songwriters: Richard Leigh / Richard C Leigh / Roger Alan Murrah

Life's Highway lyrics © Sony/ATV Music Publishing LLC

The lyrics of this song tell us life just keeps moving on down the highway whether we like it or not. The sun comes up, and the sun goes down, and we have no control over its forward movement. We cannot stop time just because we want to savor the moment or because we feel unable to move along with it due to circumstances or events beyond our control that seem to paralyze our movement.

Glenn Miller's In the Mood was sure to pack the dance floor in the 1940s. The Weaver's Goodnight Irene signaled the dance was over in the 1950s. Couples in love and lonely hearts sang along to the Righteous Brothers' Unchained Melody in the 1960s. And John Lennon pleaded to a divided nation with Give Peace a Chance in the 1970s.

The power of music to bring memories to life makes for an effective and powerful therapy.

Memories in Music

The first time I met Ona, she was sitting in the dining room of the nursing facility. Ona was calling out, "help me, help me," which had become her mantra over the previous months as Alzheimer's disease robbed her of the ability to articulate her needs, recognize her family and remember her own name. Her son, Jason visited almost daily, and though they sat side by side, his mother was a stranger to him.

Ona had been admitted to hospice as she had shown a significant decline in recent weeks. Jason had accepted music therapy as an additional service for his mother. Music therapy is offered as an opportunity for increased communication and memory recall.

On that first day, as I sat across from Ona and Jason with my guitar, Jason shared a brief history of Ona's life. Ona had loved to dance in her youth. The song Blue Skirt Waltz was the first song Ona danced to with the man who would become her husband. Ona even made a blue skirt for herself and wore it when they danced.

As I started to play the Blue Skirt Waltz, Ona's cries of "help me" ceased, and the years gently melted away as Ona was transported back to 1946. Ona lifted her head, let out a knowing sigh, and began to sing along. She held her hands out to her son, who took them. Mother and son gently swayed, dancing together while seated side by side.

I dream of that night with you, Lady when first we met...

Jason and Ona beamed at each other. Ona's eyes sparkled as if she was 18 years old again. She appeared to be dancing a first dance at the Melody Mill dance hall where she met the love of her life and dance partner of 65 years. Jason glimpsed the mother he remembered who laughed and sang, whose life was full, whose heart was young, and who remembered.

We danced in a world of blue, how could my heart forget...

I held the music steady and kept the waltz moving to provide space and support for this mother-and-son reunion.

Blue were your eyes, and blue were the skies, just like the blue skirt you wore...

The three of us continued to meet for music therapy sessions until the day Ona's condition changed. Jason and I sat vigil at her bedside and, once again, sang the song she loved.

Come back, blue lady, come back, don't be blue anymore.

While dementia had taken away the usual form of communication between mother and son, music brought them together in a whole new way. Jason was at Ona's bedside when she died, and he sang to her. At the time of her death, he envisioned his mother letting go of his hand to take the hand of her husband to continue the dance they had started long ago.

(Music Therapist)

"Oh, Danny Boy"

This is the story of Daniel. Not his life story but his death story: specifically, the last hour of Daniel's quiet, beautiful life.

I was Daniel's hospice music therapist. Dan loved music. He had a history of a brain injury years earlier. I don't know if he loved music his whole life or if it became really important for him after his injury. He wasn't able to fill in much of the story of his life due to memory loss.

He never remembered me from one visit to another. Each time I came into his room at the nursing home, his whole being lit up, and he would smile from ear to ear. It was all new each time. He would see the guitar on my back or the little Celtic lap harp I would bring. He could strum the harp and would ask about the instrument and want to hear it played. Daniel would close his eyes and hold his breath, then let it out slowly in an "ah" of wonder. It seemed his heart, soul, and the very cells that made up Daniel were responding to the vibrations. Then, he would cry. The tears were a mixture of happy and sad tears. He wouldn't know which or why but the music struck a chord with Daniel, and his emotions would flow.

The most excited I had seen Daniel get was when I came to visit when I brought my Celtic lap harp. He loved the structure of it, the beauty of the wood, and the sound. I only needed to take the harp out of its bag, and Daniel would begin crying. "Would you play it?" He would ask. We always ended our visits with his special song, "Danny Boy." "That's just for me," he would say.

I was blessed to be present at the moment Daniel died. Daniel did not have a family to be at his side, but volunteers were there with him. One of the wonderful, dedicated volunteers was holding Daniel's hand. The hospice nurse and another volunteer joined us as we all shared stories of Daniel and what a difference he made in our lives and the world. We promised him he would not be alone during this part of his journey. His breathing began to change as I played the harp strings, and it was during the song "Danny Boy" that Daniel took his last, peaceful breath, surrounded by his hospice family. We thanked Daniel for allowing us to be witnesses to this sacred time of passing. There is a line in Danny Boy: "It's you, it's you must go, and I must bide."

That was Daniel's goodbye to us. It was his turn this time. I imagine he entered his new life even more full of wonder and awe than he was in this one.

(Music Therapist)

Oh Danny Boy
Daniel O'Donnell

The pipes, the pipes are calling

From glen to glen and down the mountain side

The summer's gone

And all the flowers are dying

'Tis you, 'tis you must go

And I must bide

But come ye back when summer's in the meadow

Or when the valley's hushed

And white with snow

'Tis I'll be here in sunshine or in shadow

Oh Danny Boy, oh Danny Boy

I love you so

And if ye come

When all the flowers are dying

If I am dead as dead, I, well, may be

You'll come and find

The place where I am lying

You'll kneel and say an Ave there for me

And I shall hear though soft you tread above me

And all my grave will warmer, sweeter be

Then you will kneel

And whisper that you love me

And I shall sleep in peace until you come to me

Songwriters: Donald Michael Kasen, Frederick Edward Weatherly.

103

You've Got a Friend

The hospice nurse was scheduled to visit Bryan, a young man who had Alzheimer's. She was anxious to meet him as she had just read the book "Still Alive" which is a novel telling the story of early-onset Alzheimer's Disease from the patient's perspective. Bryan had been an architect of golf courses and had received awards from all over the world. His disease had progressed to the point where he had lost his ability to even smile, and he had become a resident at a nursing home. But he was "still alive" in his failing body. The hospice nurse entered Bryan's room at the nursing home and found him sleeping in his wheelchair. She didn't want to awaken him, so she waited patiently and made herself comfortable. She hoped to familiarize herself a little better with this intriguing young man as she looked over his CD collection of music, mostly from the 60s and 70s. She decided to choose one selection, "James Taylors Greatest Hits", and proceeded to get to know Bryan a little better as she looked through some photo albums that were lying out on his dresser while listening to James Taylor.

The soft music was comforting and happened to bring Bryan gently out of his sleep. Wanting to break the ice with conversation and knowing of his impressive history with golf courses, she asked him, "Do you know what I say about golf?" His face lit up as I'm sure he thought he had a fellow lover of golf to talk with. "What?" He asked. "Public humiliation!" She replied. A broad smile came across his face even though his hopes for a golf conversation may have been dashed. A smile from someone who had been unable to smile for some time. What a gift it was to bring an expressive smile to this face that had for so long had no reason to smile. And perhaps quite by chance, the song they were hearing at the time was "You've Got A Friend". Coincidence. I think not. A special moment, I think so. When hospice comes to visit, you've got a friend for sure.

(Hospice nurse)

I Am OK

My 54-year-old male patient with lung cancer had been experiencing denial throughout the entire time he was in our hospice program. Often on my visits, he would say, "I'm going to be OK." His condition changed rather quickly, and as I was talking to him, he said, "I'm going to be OK". Knowing that he was dying, I asked him what he meant, and he said, "I know I'm dying, but I am OK.

(Hospice nurse)

Drumming His Way Home
10-24-55 to 1-8-2014

Guy was a gifted musician and had been playing drums in different bands from the time he was 13 years old. His band playing was mostly in smoky bars all his life. Guy was what you might call a bit of a "rough rider" or from the "wrong side of the tracks". He had a wildly funny and unique sense of humor. He was one never to laugh at his own jokes. He enjoyed watching others react when they finally caught on to his dry wit. Guy had changed his ways before I met him. However, because of his "rowdy" former life, he never felt worthy of having a relationship with the Lord and distanced himself from any formal religion or worship. I had grown up in a faith tradition that I was committed to, and we sent our children to their schools. Guy would attend services for special occasions, such as holidays and any events our children were involved in through school. Over the years, I started attending another church because our youngest daughter was attending youth group there and was starting to learn about the Bible. I wanted to know too about this book that I had never explored.

As in many marriages, ours had become one that was floating on very rough waters. I had placed my children above my relationship with Guy. We had major communication problems, and one Sunday afternoon in November of 2009, we had a particularly nasty argument. I drove off in my car, and in a verbally loud, desperate plea to God, I asked Him to save our marriage. He not only restored our marriage but drew us, and especially Guy, closer to Him. For the first time, Guy started attending services regularly with me. Our pastor, knowing he was a drummer, even convinced him to play in the church band. I was thrilled, to say the least! He also agreed to attend small group bible study with other couples in the church. Those friends proved invaluable to us after Guy received his diagnosis of stage 4 lung cancer in July 2012. During our last Christmas together, they even gave us a personal Christmas caroling session in our home.

Guy was attending church and participating in the church community, but he still did not accept the free gift of salvation Jesus has offered to all of us. Shortly after the diagnosis, the pastor was one of the first persons who met with us and talked to Guy. He was able to admit to the pastor that he had never really prayed before because he never felt worthy. At that visit, he said for the first time in his life, he prayed for God's forgiveness and fully accepted His grace and mercy through His son, Jesus Christ. He said he had always felt "too bad" to have a personal relationship with Jesus. Whereas I always felt I was "good enough" to make the cut to heaven. PRIDE! Both of us were in equal need of a savior. It was that day that Guy crossed over the line in his faith life and fully accepted Jesus, his grace, and forgiveness into his heart. He accepted the free gift of salvation that so many are afraid to do because they feel they are "too bad" or, like Guy, "not good enough". This was the most joyous day of seeing him cross that line of faith.

He would walk the flood wall in our town each day, communicating with his Lord and Savior, which brought about a feeling of peace and hope he had never known until he was unable due to the progression of cancer. We were able to enjoy every day for a year and a half. Our four children were great with visiting and spending time with their dad. We all traveled to California and drove up Highway 1 to Oregon through the great generosity of family and friends. This was something Guy had always wanted to do.

He continued with church activities and playing in the church band when he felt well enough. I learned to slow down, not sweat the small stuff, and be content to just sit with my husband, who loved and adored me more than I ever deserved. Best of all, we read the Bible together and other books on God and eternity with Him. Guy continued his fight against cancer, and one evening we were sitting on our deck with a friend, praying. Guy prayed out loud for the first time, asking God to please heal him, but that he would accept whatever God's will was for him. That gave me peace and hope that's hard to explain.

He was struggling with the diagnosis but doing as well as could be expected and trying to appreciate each day. He was getting progressively worse, however, and on December 9, 2013, he was barely able to walk to the car. He was admitted to the hospital with a collapsed lung due to stage 4 of his lung disease. His oncologist said that he could not recommend any further treatment that would be effective due to his weakened condition. That news and the recommendation that he go to hospice took the little wind left out of our sails. The doctor said getting hospice would help with symptom management and pain control and should improve his quality of life. It was the best option available. That day in December will forever bring sad memories.

Next came the difficult task of telling our four children, three of whom lived away from home. Two were living out of town, and we told them to wait until the following day due to the prediction of a raging nasty snowstorm that was coming. Our middle daughter ignored me as she had done once or twice before (ha) and drove 70 miles home from the town where she was in college. The Lord was surely with her during that treacherous drive, and Guy was happy to see her. Our son, wife, and grandson lived three hours away and arrived the following day. After meeting with the hospice team and being assigned our nurse, we were sent home.

Later that afternoon, we all gathered with the hospice nurse in the den of our home where Guy spent all his time. Our daughter and her husband (who had just lost his father to cancer a year earlier) and our two other daughters heard their dad say for the first time that he was not going to be able to beat this cancer. We were all crying with the heaviness of this realization and what it meant to us. We were crying and hugging like we hadn't done before. The nurse joined right in, and at one point, Guy lifted his head and said through his tears, "how can you do this job?" She responded by saying through her own tears that she could carry the intense love she felt in the room home with her to her own family. That won us over. She was a great fit, and she understood and appreciated Guy's sense of humor. She had even followed some of his old bands.

Initially, Guy rallied on hospice care when they started him on prednisone and made adjustments to his plan of care. He was eating, joking, and loving the massages from the massage therapist. Guy's sister would come over often and cook up some "scrambles", a dish they enjoyed as kids growing up. A particularly favorite night was when our son decided to buy lobster, his dad's favorite. The whole family came, and we enjoyed a wonderful lobster fest! Guy's favorite place to vacation was Florida, and he wanted to go there and see the ocean one more time. Hospice agreed to help set things up in Florida, and it gave Guy something to look forward to.

Our days were spent together, watching old TV shows like Andy Griffith, reading the Bible or other Christian books like "Heaven Is For Real," and visiting with our children, family, friends, and the staff from hospice. He looked forward to his hospice nurse coming, the massage therapist, and anyone who would show up at our door.

On Monday, January 7th, which happened to be the week we had planned to go to Florida, I decided to go to work for half a day because our oldest daughter said she would stay with her dad all day. At 2 pm, I called Guy to see how he was doing, and he said, "Girl (my nickname), I'm a bit out of breath. Could you come home? My daughter hadn't noticed because instead of panicking, as I would have, my husband got really calm and quiet when he was struggling. I left work immediately and headed for home, about 25 miles away. Our daughter had called the hospice nurse, and she was in our home by the time I got home. He was deteriorating quickly, and she called for another hospice nurse for backup.

One of my best friends happened to be in town and stopped by. She was a God-send for me. Another good friend came in too. I called our son, who was three hours away, and my parents, who were a short distance away and very close cousins of Guys. As people started arriving at our home, Guy stated three times, "I'm not going anywhere." Our son told him he heard there was a party and he wasn't going to miss it. Guy still didn't want to die. His breathing was getting more labored, and he was struggling. He was given medications to help calm him, and we were all with him through the night.

We told Guy that his favorite hospice nurse would be coming, as well as our Pastor, at 8:00 am the next morning. I finally had my kids try to lay down around 4 am. I stayed in the den with Guy as I usually did, on the couch close to him. He was in the recliner. At about 7:30 am, his breathing became very quiet, and my friend who was staying with us told me to gather the kids. The kids were all in the room when the hospice nurse and pastor arrived at 8 am. After the hospice nurse checked him, our pastor moved in and held his hands, and prayed, saying God is waiting to welcome him into His kingdom, and he ended by quoting Psalm 150:4, 5, "praise him with the tambourine and dancing, praise him with the strings and flute, praise him with the clash of cymbals, praise him with resounding cymbals.

Being the great drummer he was, Guy listened to his final earthly instructions and took his last breath. It was peaceful; it was beautiful, and it was the saddest day of our lives. It certainly was made easier by the loving care and support of family, friends, co-workers, and the hospice team. I know without a doubt that Guy is with his Lord and Savior, not because he thought he was a good person, but because he admitted he wasn't and accepted the gift of eternal life through the sacrifice of Christ on the cross. He would be the first to say, don't wait until you have cancer to begin a personal relationship with Jesus Christ. Our only way to heaven. My middle daughter, through her tears, said, "It's better to have your dad die in his 50s knowing the Lord than to live till 99 and not know the Lord."

2 Corinthians 4:16-18

There for, we do not lose heart,

Though outwardly, we are wasting away,

Yet inwardly, we are being renewed day by day.

For our light and momentary troubles

Are achieving for us an eternal glory

That far outweighs them all.

So, we fix our eyes not on what is seen,

But on what is unseen.

For what is seen is temporary,

But what is unseen is eternal.

(Wife of hospice patient)

Humor Sets the Stage

People don't change because they receive a terminal diagnosis. If they were quiet, sensitive, outgoing, or enjoyed the humor in their life, that continues. Whatever their individual characteristics or personality was like, that continues, and it is refreshing to see the people we serve continue to enjoy small moments that can bring some humor to their days.

Teasing and Tricks

Mr. R. was a widow and a funny man who had just recently received a diagnosis of lung cancer. He was also a talker. I am a talker, and I could barely get a word in. He was admitted to our hospice program, and my visits started.

I always wondered when I first met a patient if I would be the right fit for them. Would I be the best person who could offer something beyond the expected symptom management, comfort, and support? I always trusted that God would put me where I needed to be. I think I was the right fit for Mr. R.

He had one local daughter and two daughters that lived a distance away. One in the south and one toward the southeastern part of the country. Without much explanation, he conveyed that he had the desire to get these three daughters together once again. It had been a long time since they were all together. He was looking for a time to share and bond once again. This was important to him. Distance has a way of breaking down some of those close bonds we felt when we were younger and growing up together. He wanted to make sure this bond between his girls was renewed. It became a deep but almost unspoken desire before he died.

As I said, he was a talker and full of mischievous energy, proclaiming to enjoy every minute of life till the end. He never voiced any anger or sadness about his current situation and the terminal diagnosis. He seemed to embrace the fullness of life ahead of him rather than focus on the negatives he was facing. We had become more comfortable with each visit, and I was starting to understand and appreciate his great sense of humor. He continued to talk, talk, and talk. I can't say for sure if it was nervous energy or just his personality, but he was a talker.

I'd like to think I'm pretty good at reading people, and I began to feel a real comfort with him. So one day, when I was making my visit, I decided to test his sense of humor. I felt certain he would be a good sport about it. As I began my assessment, including listening to his heart and lung sounds, I appeared to be doing a more thorough job, and it took me more time than usual. He knew he had to be quiet during the assessment so I could clearly hear his heart and lung sounds. He was handling his imposed silence quite well, I thought. As I finished, I decided I needed to be honest with him. So I confessed to him that I didn't actually need all that time for the assessment, but I was just trying to see how long he could keep quiet. That was it. It cemented our relationship. As I remember, I think he was a little speechless when I made my confession. Now the game was on. I met him at his level, and he appreciated that. We go where they lead us. It is their journey.

With my ongoing visits and as time passed, we did have conversations that became more serious as his disease progressed. It became increasingly apparent he had this deep desire to have all three of his daughters together. The plan was for all of them to gather together at the home of one of the daughters who lived in the south. He was happily anticipating this reunion with all of them being together again.

He was very open and forthcoming about his illness and was willing to share about coping with the disease and terminal illness. We were going to help him tell the story of his illness and reconnect with his daughters. It was something he wanted to do. He had a relative who worked in media and created presentations for public education. They were going to come and record his story and videotape the sendoff and capture the reunion story to share with others. He was aware of the need to get this done soon as his prognosis was not the best. We planned to help make this happen for him as soon as possible. We were looking at making arrangements with him to get airline tickets for himself and the local daughter. However, he seemed to be dragging his feet. Whenever I asked if he'd purchased the tickets, he was always going to get them "next week".

People often have an instinct about what's happening to them. He must have sensed more than even he realized because there was a dramatic turn in the course of his illness before he was able to purchase the tickets, and he quickly became bed-bound. This family reunion he had so desired with his daughters was not likely to happen.

With this decline, the out-of-town daughters were updated, and they made arrangements to come home to help with caregiving for their father. Adjustments were made to his Plan of Care for his improved comfort, and a hospital bed was set up in the home. Instructions were provided for the daughters regarding his care, with repeated instructions to call our "on-call" nurse, who was available 24/7 if there were any questions. The girls were united in caring for their dad, and they fully embraced this newly offered gift of caregiving for him. They became very focused on doing it right for him. One night they started to search the internet when they thought of something they wanted to know. For some reason, they did not call the hospice "on-call" nurse as they had been instructed. They needed to do this for their dad as much on their own as possible. It became their gift to him.

During this time, he was becoming less responsive, and the girls were truly doing their best to provide the care he needed. I tell families that care received at the end of life is so important, and the hands that provide that care are special hands. It is even more special when those hands are family because the hands are also loving hands. That does make a difference. Anything they did for their dad was provided by loving hands which could never be anything but the best for him.

They were doing a very good job, but knowing their dad as they did, they confessed to him that they felt they probably weren't doing as good a job as their mother would have. At that moment, his humorous nature mustered the energy to respond to them, "You're darn right about that," which brought a chuckle to all three girls. He never did get to make the trip which he somehow must have known he wouldn't be able to do. The three daughters he so desperately wanted to bring together were in his home now, knitting together an even deeper bond as they became united in this beautiful effort of caring for their father. No trip could have compared to the connection these girls experienced in those days caring for their dear dad. The testimony of love for a father was very evident throughout his final days. I know being cared for by his daughters in his home during his journey to the next world was greater than any trip he could have taken with his local daughter to see the other two girls. He was a father blessed by unlikely circumstances.

Also noteworthy and so like this man's personality is a story the daughters related to us during their days with their dad. Wanting to offer support in every aspect of life, we often ask whether all their needs are being met, physical, psycho-social, emotional, and spiritual. He decided he would like a visit from the pastor of his local church, who just happened to be newly ordained and quite young. The time was set up, and the appointed day arrived. The pastor arrived, and the girls left the room so their dad could have some private time with the priest. The pastor seemed fine when he arrived, but as the visit concluded and he was ready to leave, the girls noted he seemed different, even a little distressed. They came to find out that during the time their fun-loving father had been talking with the priest, his hands entwined with the priest as he was providing support to Mr. R... something unexpected happened. In this very solemn moment, suddenly, the patient became limp, his hand dropped from the priest's grasp, and it appeared he had died right there in the pastor's presence. The priest was obviously distraught at this sudden turn of events before his very eyes. After only a few moments, which must have felt like forever to the priest, the patient opened his eyes and quickly said to the priest, "Gotcha, didn't I?" He was playing tricks, yet as he was slipping nearer to the end of his life. What a guy. I will never forget him. And I don't think the priest will either.

(Hospice nurse)

Bring Your Humor

Mrs. D was widowed and in her 90s and still able to live in her own home alone when she received her terminal diagnosis. Having lived many years and having raised a large family, she was very skilled at many things in life. One of her specialties was making pies. She had stacks of mini pie tins so she could make a special individual pie for each grandchild when they came to visit. Her many children were scattered across the area, and some lived many miles away. When she was admitted to hospice care, some of the daughters came to be with her and help in her care as needed. There was always witty banter happening when I would come to visit. But there was also an air of heaviness as the daughter's impending sense of loss with their mother's illness and the decline was becoming more apparent.

Each visit would end up around the kitchen table, with the daughters sharing coffee and discussing what was best for mom when, in truth, mom knew what was best for her. Mrs. D required a procedure every other day to drain the fluid from around her lungs. It wasn't particularly uncomfortable but required time and caused the daughters some anxiety as they were unfamiliar with this medical intervention.

After many weeks of frequent visits, the conversations

became easier, light, and more comfortable as we got to know each other better. Trust was building, and there was a sense the mom loved the family being present, even as they became somewhat overprotective in their loving way. At one visit, feeling very comfortable in everyone's presence, the girls recognized they had been so focused on mom's condition and care that they had failed to offer me their usual morning coffee as we sat together at their table. They made their apologies, and I wasn't certain I wanted or needed a cup of coffee at that moment.

Sometimes, something comes out of my mouth, and I wonder how that happened. But I felt very comfortable with this family, and conversations had become very familiar and relaxed. At that very moment, I declined the coffee and unwittingly said, "Maybe next time, it will be fresher then." I was shocked at my bold rudeness, as the comment elicited big laughs from the daughters as well as the mom, who were all very good-spirited. I knew we had been on solid ground, but I apologized profusely, which made them laugh even more. Feeling deeply sad that I had "over-stepped" my boundaries with them, I apologized to the mom and said, "I am so very sorry. I will never do that again. You probably won't want me to come back". Mom took my hand and looked me straight in the eye, and with the most sincere words, said, "No, you come back, and bring your humor." I have chills remembering how this faux pas brought a little lightheartedness when this lady needed it. It is never our intention to offend anyone, but sometimes the moment presents itself with humor, and we are graced with the kindness of those we serve, and it turns out okay. I always hoped and prayed that when a patient is assigned to me, I will be the right "fit" for them. Then something like this happens, and we know we are where we are supposed to be, doing what we are meant to do.

(Hospice nurse)

Simple Pleasures, Please

Bud was in his late 80s and being cared for by a local home care agency. He was diagnosed with end-stage heart disease and confined to his home to qualify for home care services. The nurses regularly came to assess and direct his care. It was spring, and the home care nurse had been in for her usual assessment recently. His family had just gathered and celebrated Easter, and Bud was sharing how he enjoyed the celebration with all the festive food, including ham. He shared how the home care nurse had just admonished him for the breach in his cardiac diet.

His family had been considering hospice care for him, but it was not encouraged by his primary physician. They now decided they would give hospice care a try. The hospice informational meeting was held with the family present as hospice staff explained all the aspects of care and the benefits of using hospice for Bud's care.

As Bud's primary nurse, on my first visit to the home, I took the time to assure Bud that he could eat and drink anything he wanted. He paused, looked at me, and asked, "What did you say?" I repeated the encouragement that he could eat and drink whatever he wanted. We would not be placing any restrictions on his diet. Bud was already not eating and drinking his normal intake as he had in the past due to his changing health. I looked at him and repeated,

"You can eat and drink anything you want." I further explained, "We are not here to take things away from you but to bring things to you and help you enjoy and make each day the best it can be. That includes eating whatever you want." He looked at his family, who were seated nearby, and said, "Did you hear that?" Bud had really only wanted to enjoy a piece of bacon, or ham, or a highball one a week. How could anyone admonish him for such simple pleasures? They were making memories with these precious moments.

The weeks rolled on, and we continued to provide support and encouragement to Bud, his wife, and their devoted family. During the weeks we were able to serve Bud, he was able to get out to a surprise birthday party for one of his sons, he was able to attend a family wedding, and he was even able to take a car ride with his adult children and go through the drive-up at McDonald's so he could buy them an ice cream cone like he had done when they were kids. Simple pleasures.

My favorite memory of Bud was one that revealed his great sense of humor. He had a Pleur-X drain implanted in his chest to drain the fluid accumulation around his lungs resulting from his disease. On the first day I was to drain his catheter, his daughter, who is a friend and also a nurse, suggested that dad lay down on his bed for the procedure. I assured them I could perform the procedure wherever it was comfortable for him, and he could remain seated wherever he was for the drainage. The daughter thought it best for dad to lay down, so we proceeded to his bedroom, and he sat down on the bed and then found a comfortable position lying down. The daughter climbed onto the bed beside him for support. I was essentially in bed to get close enough to do the procedure. And his cardiac nurse, who happened to be present during the visit, was leaning over the edge of the bed in support of Bud as well. Bud's wife was standing off to the side, patiently waiting for this "ominous" procedure to happen as these three women hovered over her beloved husband. At that moment, to our surprise, Bud simply stated, "I don't think I can ever remember being in bed with three women before", at which time all of us burst out laughing. To add to the light moment, I quickly added, "Well, if you are going to tell people about being in bed with three women, make sure you tell them that all three of the women had smiles on their faces." Bud created a beautiful and humorous moment that I will never forget.

(Hospice nurse)

People don't change because they receive a terminal or life-limiting diagnosis. The traits and characteristics that made them the person they are remain with them to the end.

They only want and need to be assured that those who journey with them will accept them for who they are and also honor how they live their life. Humor can be an essential and integral part of coping needed to endure the journey. We meet them where they are in their life, honoring and respecting who they are, who they have been, and how they choose to finish their journey.

I love it when humor comes through. It lightens a heavy load for many. There are so many unexpected gifts received by those of us who journey with these incredible people who allow us into their lives when they are most vulnerable. We celebrate with them all that they are and, many times, are surprised and humbled by the gifts we receive on the journey.

(Hospice nurse)

I've learned that people will forget what you said, people will forget what you did, but people will never forget how you made them feel.

Maya Angelou

I Think It's A Hangover

Hazel was a feisty little lady who had lived fully during her 100 years of life. As her niece, I was always impressed with Hazel. She seemed enduring, loving, and always up for a good laugh. Hazel managed to live in her own home until about 18 months before her death. Two years before, she had fallen in her home and fractured her femur, requiring surgery and follow-up rehab in a skilled care facility. She recovered and managed to return to her home, where she had lived for most of those 100 years. In the months following her fracture and rehab, she contracted pneumonia five times. With each episode, she was losing some ground. She was feisty enough to continue to remain in her home with some additional contracted help checking in on her.

I would frequently joke with Hazel that she and I were the only two people in the city with the same last name, both of us acquiring the name by marriage. Our local paper had in the past posted a "police beat" section, mentioning those members of the community who had found themselves in trouble with the law. I joked with her that if that name ended up in the "police beat" section of the paper, it was either her or me. She would laugh, knowing neither of us would likely end up in that section of the paper. She always enjoyed a good laugh and was able to find the lighthearted side to any situation.

During one of her hospitalizations, after which the gentleman who generally checked on her had found her on the floor in the bathroom, she remarked she had fallen, and unfortunately, her lifeline wrist alert band was caught under her. She was unable to reach it to call for help. She went on to tell me she had laid on the bathroom floor for nearly 24 hours before someone finally arrived to find her in this arduous predicament. During that time, she had gotten thirsty, and in her ever-problem-solving mode, she thought if she could just wriggle her way close enough to the stool, she might be able to relieve her thirst, just like dogs do. Oh, Hazel! Now that's what you call making the best of a bad situation.

Her humor never wavered, and she was always excited about a visit as her family lived miles away from her. She had been transported from her home by ambulance multiple times and was now residing permanently in the nursing home. On one such return by medical transport from the hospital back to her nursing home room, my grandson and I were standing outside the room as they were getting her moved from the transport cart and settled in her bed. My grandson and I could overhear her admonish the transport attendant to make sure "you don't drop me" as they transferred her from the cart to the bed.

With her frequent hospitalizations from pneumonia and

decreasing stamina and functional ability, she was deemed appropriate and admitted to the hospice program. During one of my visits to her in the nursing home, I asked if she'd like to go back to see her home one last time.

She had always been an avid Chicago Cubs baseball fan and followed her beloved team closely. Fortunately for her, they had just won the World Series. We worked at making arrangements to get her home one last time, but she was now wheelchair-bound, and there were several steps into her house. Enlisting the support and services of a local community outreach program to help with setting up a temporary ramp to accommodate her wheelchair for access to the house, the date was set. The volunteer who helped with setting up the ramp became aware of Hazel's dedication to her favorite baseball team, and he generously brought a Win Flag for this devoted fan. There are so many good people in this world, and we encountered many of them on this adventure for Hazel.

She entered her home and proceeded to be wheeled into each of the rooms for one last opportunity to cherish what this home and each room had meant to her throughout her life. Rooms where she raised her children and provided a loving environment for all who entered her door. She proceeded to the kitchen, where she sat at the table, and as her daughter noted, "she was holding court" for all those present as she reminisced about many fond moments in her life. She returned to the nursing home with a content heart, having now bid farewell to her beloved home.

She continued a steady, slow decline, and on one of my visits, I noted she had not even gotten out of bed. It was already 1 pm, and that was unusual for her. Putting on my nursing hat, I proceeded to quiz her as to why she wasn't feeling well enough to get up. Was she having pain, nausea, or discomfort of any kind? She did not offer any explanation and just remained snugly tucked into her cozy bed. I sat with her, and eventually, the nurse came in and began the same inquiry into why she was not getting up. She was slow in responding, but in her typical humorous fashion, she rolled toward us and looked up into the nurse's eyes, and glibly said, "I think it's a hangover." This woman's spirit never faltered, even if it seemed stalled at times.

She was also an avid fan of the TV show Blue Bloods and specifically Tom Selleck. She had several autographed photos of him in her room, compliments of family and friends who wanted to do something special for this adorable lady. When she got moved from one room to another, she always made sure those pictures were in a prominent place where she could look at her "love".

Whenever my grandson from out of town would visit me, I made sure we'd go see Aunt Hazel because just the sight of him would make her eyes light up. It happened to be Thanksgiving weekend, and with my grandson home, we went to see Aunt Hazel, who was showing serious signs of decline. During our visit, she made sure to get her hugs from him and lovingly gave him a little knick-knack from the stash of little treasures that she still possessed. She loved him so, and he brightened her world when he was present. It was always such a joy to spend time with her, and my grandson will always remember this treasured aunt. She was able to see her beloved baseball team capture the World Series and get home for one last visit, and now she could also find her way home to the next place. She died peacefully, and before she was taken by the funeral home, the staff at the nursing home tucked the pictures of Tom Selleck, her "love", neatly on the pillow beside her head. She has left an indelible imprint on my life and heart and has shown many of us how to hang onto humor and love every moment of life right up to the very end. God bless you and rest in peace, my dear Aunt Hazel.

(Hospice nurse)

More Stories
A Life Well Lived

When I first met Beau, I had no idea how that quote would describe the final journey of his life. To meet and get to know Beau was to instantly enjoy his company. Beau was an affable and comedic soul – quick to smile, laugh or strike up a conversation with anyone willing to listen. He had a great voice, thoroughly enjoyed his time with our music therapist, and loved talking about sports. He was a Twins baseball fan, and he loved bowling. I did not realize that striking up a conversation with Beau about bowling would lead us to the one life goal Beau had left to accomplish on his bucket list. Beau wasn't just a bowler; he lived bowling for over 45 years.

He had taught many people the fine sport of bowling over the years. He attended the Brunswick School of Bowling and began teaching locally to anyone who wanted to play the sport he loved. He was a member of the American Bowling Congress and Local Bowling Association, and he had started numerous leagues and traveling teams. His personal accomplishments included three 300 games, thirty league championships, an 800 series, and nearly one hundred 700 series.

By the time I met Beau, he was no longer bowling. His body was not able to engage physically in the sport he loved so much. He handled it with the same shrugging smile and tolerance he had when faced with a 7-10 split. From our initial visits, it became apparent that Beau's last bowling desire was to attend his induction ceremony into the Local Bowling Hall of Fame. This was Beau's goal, and our goal is to help our patients live fully until they die. We would do everything possible to help him achieve this goal.

Our hospice team developed a plan that helped manage his symptoms and allowed him to participate fully in his daily activities. With the team effort of hospice, we were able to help this bowling star be welcomed into this unique and prestigious fraternity by all the members of the Local Bowling Hall of Fame, along with his protégé Buck and friend Donald. He received the admiration of his peers, and there wasn't a dry eye in the place as those who had known him through the years were able to honor him for his bowling accomplishments and also his personal character. He received a collection of photos to remember this most important moment in his life. The smile on his face was evidence of how important this accomplishment was to him. Although his memory began to fade quickly, the honor remained a sweet memory for him. He died peacefully nearly one month to the day following his induction. This was a fitting end to a life well-lived.

(Hospice nurse)

Another Life Well Lived

Miriam was a lady with a very strong faith and loved her family more than anything. She was beautiful, kind, strong, caring, and classy in every way, and gifted with a talent for art. Their home was evidence of her talent in displaying her amazing artwork. She was committed to her husband and four children despite having been diagnosed with breast cancer 11 years earlier. Her resolve to live every moment of life despite her cancer diagnosis never wavered. Her resolve to live life fully intensified when her cancer returned.

She was now in her 40s, and as her disease progressed, she became an even stronger role model for living every moment of life for her family and all who knew her. In the years since her original diagnosis, she attended her children's athletic games, including designing T-shirts for her son's high school baseball team's state appearance. She would attend every sporting event, including those that required travel, as she insisted on supporting her family no matter what she was feeling. She traveled to play-off games and would not miss a senior night with her son. She continued to meet regularly with her ladies' church group.

She accomplished a personal goal of opening an art gallery with paintings and photography and would take and fulfill orders received after the gallery opening. She was involved in her children's school activities, never missing her role in registering the children for school or preparing them for college life.

As her disease progressed and signs of her decline became more and more evident, she insisted the family plan a several-day vacation to a Chicago Cubs game. The day came, and they were headed for Chicago. They were able to enjoy the game, walk on the beach and make the most of their family time together. She would not shrink from any opportunity to help her family live the life she wanted for them. Upon return from their Chicago trip, which had been very draining for her, she was fatigued and weak but insisted on playing cards with family members that evening.

Around midnight that night, her husband noticed her breathing had changed and called the children to be at her side. She died very peacefully with her family at her side, having filled her last day with the most wonderful family time she could.

She was so driven to give her family the best; she even encouraged them to take advantage of a once-in-a-lifetime opportunity for a trip to South America with her son's basketball team after she was no longer here. The family did make the trip in her honor. She was also the inspiration for a benefit to raise money for breast cancer at her children's high school. The school gym was packed during the sporting event and inspired support from the opposing team as they recognized the spirit and dedication this extraordinary woman so exemplified.

This woman of strength will continue to be an inspiration to many and leaves a legacy of how to live life to the very fullest right up to the last breath. A great lesson for all of us. She will live on in the memory of many.

(Hospice nurse)

Build a Bed

I was working a weekend shift "on call" and visiting a patient in an Assisted Living facility in a nearby town. The need for the visit on the weekend was due to the changes that were happening with the patient. The patient's decline was increasing, and upon my visit, it was determined the patient would benefit from having a hospital bed. We contract for larger pieces of medical equipment and are always at the mercy of the providers for availability and service to secure the needed pieces of equipment.

I called one of our local Durable Medical Equipment providers. Yes, they had a bed, but the people who routinely do the delivery and set-up of the equipment were not available. I was talking to someone from the equipment department, but she was not familiar with the set-up of equipment. She failed to let me know that little piece of information when she assured me the bed would be delivered. I returned to the office to pick up the bedding we would need to prepare the bed for the patient.

I arrived back at the patient's apartment in the Assisted Living Facility at the appointed time when the bed was to arrive. The DME attendant was very accommodating in bringing in the bed pieces and getting them into the room where the bed was to be set up. As she progressed in laying out the pieces of equipment, it became more apparent that she wasn't in her comfort zone with this task. She continued diligently placing the pieces in the proper order and began assembling the bed. She was performing this unfamiliar task without concern, complaint, or any obvious stress. I was in the room, and when she finally had the bed assembled and ready for the linens, she confided to me that this wasn't among her typical assigned duties. She was more proficient in the area of respiratory equipment.

I had to take a moment to comprehend what had actually happened. It was a weekend, it was on call, and here was a lady who was not even an employee of our hospice. She had gone above and beyond to provide not only equipment unfamiliar to her, but she struggled to make sure it was set up correctly and available for the comfort of our patient. This lady went above and beyond to help us live out the mission statement of our agency of caring for the dying. I will never forget the kind and generous spirit of this lady who made me and our hospice look good that day. Her gift to the patient and our hospice was immeasurable. God Bless this beautiful lady.

(Hospice nurse)

A Beer, Please

Rosie was a delightful, fun-filled lady. She had met the love of her life, Jake, when they were young, and they hit it off from the start. They loved to dance and were experts at it. They spent many a night dancing until the music stopped. She loved to bowl as much as she loved dancing and set many bowling records within her bowling community.

Rosie was admitted to hospice, and my visits began. Each visit became more and more enjoyable as I got to know Rosie and Jake better. Medical issues and concerns were addressed, and adjustments were made to her Plan of Care for comfort as she desired. We would then proceed to the light banter we enjoyed as I became increasingly familiar with this couple, who were still so obviously in love. It began to feel like going home every time I stepped into their house.

Rosie started showing signs of decline, and a hospital bed was ordered and set up, and we got Rosie settled into bed in the middle of their living room. She was a stylish lady with a little sass, and it seemed appropriate that she should occupy the center of their home despite the circumstances that brought her to this unusual place of prominence. Wanting to make her transition to this new location less demoralizing and also realizing she would most likely remain in this bed for the remainder of her days, I asked her if there was anything she might like or want when I came next. Never knowing what people might answer, we are open to providing whatever is within our power if it might give them a lift or lighten their load. Without hesitation, Rosie answered, "Well, I would like a beer." That sounded more than reasonable, but wanting to make sure I accommodated her request, I asked her what kind of beer she would like. "A Miller," she responded. No problem. I knew I could make that happen.

On my next visit, with a beer in hand and being quite proud of my ability to satisfy her simple wish, I entered the house. We got the preliminary assessment and care adjustments out of the way, and I proceeded to get the beer for her. I really was making her wish come true. Hearing the sound of the bottle cap being removed from the bottle even brought a thirst to my senses. I proceeded to dab the mouth swab into the beer to be sure we didn't cause any aspiration and placed the beer-soaked swab in her mouth. She sucked the beer off the swab, but there was no immediate reaction from her. Feeling overly confident that I had just made a grand contribution to her day, I asked her what she thought of the beer. In a very somber but revealing tone, she simply replied, "Good, but it would have been better if it had been a Lite."

Although my ego and pride had been rightfully deflated

(I should have asked more specific questions about what kind of beer) by her simple statement, I soon realized how much I appreciated this sassy lady's honest response; she still had that spunk and determination that helped her become the best dancer and lady bowler in the city. I just hope they have the right kind of beer in heaven.

(Hospice nurse)

Verna " –Life Has To Go On"

Verna (known as Veronica) was born in Boronicia, Austria, on April 16, 1910. Austria would later be divided into smaller countries. Yugoslavia was one of those countries, and Verna and her family considered Yugoslavia to be their home. According to Yugoslavian rules at the time, young men were required to serve in the armed forces for three years. Following the three years of service to his country, Verna's father, Josef, married her mother, Marta. Her father had decided to come to America in April of 1913. He came with brothers, uncles, and other relatives. When they got to America, a couple of his brothers and uncles stayed in Pennsylvania to work in the coal mines. Her father traveled on to the rural Midwest area where he worked for one of his cousins cutting trees and building a log house. He worked with his brothers-in-law, and they combined their money to send for Josef's family.

After Josef left for America, Veronica and her family lived with her maternal grandparents. She would explain, "Mom helped her parents work hard taking care of her children, Veronica, Michele, and Jonas, as well as her siblings who were small." They were happy in life, sleeping in the hay loft as the house only had three rooms. The barn was attached to the house. They had one cow and a big garden. The house was on a small hillside, and the children made their own fun rolling down the hill. Grandpa worked in a mill, and Grandma had pretty flowers all around the house. When her father sent for them to come to America, the time came for them to say goodbye to their homeland. Her mother Marta, who was only 26 years old, her sister Michele, and Veronica, who was only three, and her brother Jonas who was one, left their grandparent's home in Boronicia and sailed on the La Provence ship from Havre, Austria on October 11, 1913. Their ship was destroyed by a German U-Boat three years later. Verna would tell how saying goodbye and never seeing any of her relatives again was hard on her mother.

Marta, Michele, Veronica, and brother Jonas arrived in New York on October 18th, 1913. According to the ship log, Marta had a total of $15.00 with her when they arrived at Ellis Island. Verna recalls, "We came on the ship with Dad's cousins and were sick all the while on the ship." "Having cousins to travel with was good for us because we could not speak very good English or understand it well." She remembered the first thing they saw upon reaching America was the Statue of Liberty. They had to go through Ellis Island to enter the United States. It was very noisy, with children screaming if they became separated from their families. The children held on very tight to Marta's dress as she held little one-year-old Jonas.

Everyone was examined to make sure they were healthy

and were checked for passports. She remembers the buildings were so high, so different than in Yugoslavia. She remembers sleeping on the floor at Ellis Island, and it was there they were given American names. Marta's name was changed to Marcella. Michele was now Marion, Veronica was now Verna, Jonas was now Jack, and her last name was spelled differently as well. Her mother did not want to raise any issues about the name changes because she did not want to cause a concern that might result in them being sent back to Yugoslavia.

"After going through Ellis Island, we went by train from New York to rural Iowa." They stayed one night in New York, sleeping in the train station, and left for Chicago on the train the next day. In Chicago, they boarded a train to Iowa.

When we reached the Midwest, there was snow on the ground. We were met by a gentleman with a team of horses and a bobsled. We were all bundled up with warm blankets and arrived at my uncles home at about midnight. These wonderful people fed us and put us to bed on straw ticks on the floor. I will always cherish the memories of these wonderful people and their families. We always had enough to eat. We had potatoes and meat and fresh bread every day. The men did a lot of hunting for rabbits and squirrels. We lived with this family for five months. "I remember getting a red apple for our first Christmas in America. We started school in the spring, and it was hard because we did not speak English very well. The family we lived with spoke German. The teacher was German, and she was very nice to us."

Verna stayed in contact with this family and their descendants, attending reunions with them throughout her life. She was so grateful for their kindness when she came to America. Four more siblings would join Verna's family through the years. They moved to a two-room house, and her dad started working for the railroad. "We were very poor. A farmer sometimes gave us a 50-pound bag of cornmeal that he ground at home and also a can of milk. Dad would bring old railroad ties for use in our cook stove, which was our only heat. Sometimes Dad and Mom would saw the railroad ties in the kitchen."

"My folks never missed Mass. They only had one pair of shoes between them. One would go to early Mass and the other to late Mass. Dad made shoes for us children. We walked barefoot to school until it got too cold. Dad got his citizenship papers in 1919, and we all became citizens. I was so proud of my dad. We moved a lot and felt lucky when we found berries and nuts in the woods near our home. Dad continued to work for the railroad until we moved to a farm."

"I graduated from eighth grade in 1925 and went to high

school for one year. Then I worked for a family. Sometimes we had parties at school, and we brought box lunches. We used shoe boxes covered with wallpaper and tied with ribbon. Our boxes, with our names inside, contained two homemade buns with jelly, pickles, and a piece of cake. My sisters and I got $1.25 for our boxes."

"We couldn't date until we were 17 years old. I didn't date many guys. House parties were fun, and we would play spin the bottle, dance, eat lunch and go home. I met Francis (who was German and had been born in America) at a house party in 1927, and we got engaged on October 5th, 1929. Francis gave me a nice watch and ring to celebrate our engagement. He took me out for dinner but did not have the $1.50, so he charged it. He was only making $30.00 a month, and he had bought a Chevrolet car and was paying$15.00 a month on car payments. We were married on January 12th, 1932. The week after my wedding, my folks were sold out by the bank (foreclosed) for $220.00. Cattle, hogs, and machinery were all gone. It was sad for all of us, but we learned to deal with it. "Life has to go on." That became a saying often heard from Verna throughout the years as they learned how to survive many hardships.

Much of Verna's strength, courage, and determination were the result of her upbringing. Francis and Verna were married for 60 years and had seven children. They experienced difficult and demanding financial concerns for many years as they worked hard on their farm. Verna worked helping with the farm work, such as picking corn by hand, planting a large garden, and canning the produce from the garden. She was an excellent cook and was known for her homemade bread and coconut pies. She could take a leftover from the refrigerator and turn it into a gourmet dish. Everyone was welcomed to her home and fed before they left.

Verna grieved the loss of her husband Francis when he died on February 8th, 1992. She also lost three of her children, two of them in the same year, and a granddaughter. She was no stranger to loss. She was a woman of faith, saying her rosary daily for her children (a decade for each child and their family). Verna's life was a witness to the strength and determination she saw in her parents and family throughout her growing-up years. She passed along that same strength and determination to her family whenever she faced hardships in her life. She taught everyone how to survive challenges and trials. "Life has to go on".

Verna suffered a small stroke in 2005. She left her apartment and transferred from the hospital to the local nursing home. Everyone knew this was going to be difficult for her. Several of her family were waiting at the nursing home when she arrived. As she was wheeled into the home, she looked at all of her family, smiled, and said, "Welcome to my new home, kids," making the situation easier for her children. "Life has to go on".

Through the years at the nursing home, she nurtured her roommates and many others as they needed love and attention. She was often the last resident to go to bed at night. She enjoyed having staff come into her room in the evening and sit and visit as she shared stories about her life and opinions on issues of the day. She was very proud of her heritage and had a copy of the ship log or "Manifest of Alien Passengers for the United States of America Immigration Office at the Port of Arrival" from Ellis Island with her name on it. It was framed and hanging on the wall in her room at the nursing home. It was a symbol of the pride she had for her heritage.

Staff at the nursing home came to love her as their own family. She loved attending Mass weekly, listening to music, especially polka music, spelling contests, bowling, and dressing in costumes for Halloween parties. She was very competitive during any of the contests, whether it was a Halloween costume or bowling, but especially spelling. She kept written records of her successes in a spiral notebook at her bedside. On one of the pages in her notebook, she wrote: "thank you and bye-bye 2008."

Buying her annual calendar was significant to her and

usually happened when she went to a famous nearby apple orchard with her oldest son in October. Spending a day with her family was always special. She loved going to a park or wooded area, riding on a motorcycle with her grandson at age 98, and riding on a snowmobile at age 99. Verna was interviewed for a local news publication when she was 101-1/2. It was titled "Coming to America." She was very proud of the article. She said she felt like she was an important celebrity after it was published. She loved being called a celebrity. The author ended the article "Verna - A Lady Who Lived History."

A memorable day was when her four surviving children gathered with her in a van, and they visited all of the places she had lived through the years. Pictures of each site were taken even though things had changed through the many years. Much reminiscing, laughter, and thoughts of Francis and her three deceased children took place that day.

She loved to dance and explained her dad had taught her and her siblings how to dance so they would know how when they started dating. She danced with her four surviving children at her 100th birthday party. Celebrating parties was a big part of Verna's life, and her family enjoyed planning fun get-togethers for her. They used to tell her she had more parties than anyone else they knew. They held big celebrations for her 87th, 97th, 100th, 101st, and 102nd birthdays. On most birthdays, immediate family would take her out for dinner. The family had told her nothing was planned for her 102nd birthday. She kept asking the staff at the nursing home if they thought the family had planned anything. She would stop any staff she encountered and ask, "Do you think there's going to be a party." "Do you think they're planning a surprise?" Many staff would relate their encounter with her and the delight she would show when she would question them about any upcoming surprise party in her honor.

The morning of her 102nd birthday, she requested assistance in dressing in her nicest outfit and her pearls. She wanted to be ready just in case. She wasn't disappointed as the family did invite all of her children, grandchildren, and close friends to come to the nursing home to celebrate her 102nd birthday on April 15th, 2012. When her son wheeled her to the party room, she acted very surprised. Everyone felt she deserved an academy award for her performance. She enjoyed her day as she held the hands of each of her guests and made them feel special. Sadly, that was her last party. She died less than a month later, on May 9th, 2012.

In the days before she died, hospice had been called in to provide support and care for her. The family faithfully sat in vigil at her bedside as she became unresponsive in the days leading up to her death. She was loved by everyone at the nursing home, and she made each of them feel special. Individually staff would take the time to come see her one more time and say their last goodbyes to this lady who brought so much life with her everywhere she went. The family remembers as each staff member would come privately to her room to pay their respects one last time, and before they would leave the room, they would purposefully come to the family and tell them that Verna told each of them that they were "her favorite." She had made many "favorite" friends at the nursing home and throughout her life. Everyone was "her favorite".

How special that this lady, who had lived so much history and survived things most of us would consider hardships today, was able to make everyone she encountered in this world feel special. She never felt slighted or that she suffered any hardship too great to survive. She never lost her zest for living life to the fullest. That's a legacy that is hard to match and one that is an inspiration for all of us. I'm sure she is now enjoying every birthday in heaven, and I feel certain there is a party happening too.

(Hospice nurse and family of the patient)

Connections
What's That Smell?

The hospice volunteer lived in the same small town as the patient she was assigned to. The patient was an elderly lady whose main caregiver was her young granddaughter-in-law. In the spirit of support that often happens in small towns, the volunteer told the caregiver that if she was ever scared or needed help, she could call this volunteer anytime, night or day. The granddaughter took her up on her offer several times.

Sometimes the disease can cause an odor that might seem unpleasant, and this happened to be the case with Anna. The house was lovely, and they had candles burning, with one set in front of the statue of the Blessed Virgin Mary. The candles helped to lessen the odor throughout the house, but the room where Anna lay still had a hint of the odor.

On the morning that Anna was dying, the volunteer was called, and she remained with the family through Anna's death until the funeral home came and went. That evening the volunteer went to bed early and was reading in bed when suddenly she became aware of a very unpleasant smell. It got her attention, and she sat straight up, wondering where it could be coming from in her home. Just as quickly as she sat up, a very sweet and wonderful smell filled the room. She realized then she had been given the gift of knowing that Anna was safely home. She smiled and said aloud, "Thank you, Anna, for letting me know you made it home and you're alright."

(Hospice volunteer)

Strong Connections with Grandpa

A dear friend was in a serious traffic accident that took the life of her husband and left her physically compromised for some time after the accident, which required the family to provide care during the following months. Several months after the accident, her daughter was visiting, and she had her four-year-old daughter with her. They were sitting in the living room talking about this dear husband, father, and grandfather who had died in the accident. Without prompting, the granddaughter said, "He's here; don't you see him?" My friend said, "No, honey, I don't see him. Can you see him?" With all the innocence of a four-year-old, she said, "yeah, he's here," and she waved her hand to him. She then said, "He's light; he's not heavy. He's going to sit on my lap. But that's OK, grandma, he's light, he's not heavy. He's here. He's OK. I can see him." The friend told the little girl that she and her daughter were not able to see him. "He's not letting us see him, but you are able to see him, and I bet he wishes he could have spent more time with you. He always called you his little pip."

Some years later, this same friend was talking with another granddaughter who had not yet been born before her husband died. The little girl was quite young at this time. They were again talking about the husband, father, and grandfather who had died in this tragic accident.

Reminiscing about what he was like and what he liked to do so this little girl could better understand who her grandfather was. They had a picture of him and were showing it to the little girl. My friend told the granddaughter that she would really have loved grandpa, and she was really sad that the little girl didn't get to be here with him and get to know him. The granddaughter looked at my friend and said, "He knows me; he knows me. I met him before I came here. Didn't you know that, grandma?" She said he "was really nice grandma." In her most sincere and convincing voice, she said, "well, grandma, I knew him. I knew what he was like." She was absolutely positive about knowing a grandpa she had never met in this world.

(Hospice nurse)

Are They Really Gone

The social worker remembered many years ago being assigned to a young man who was in his 20s and dying. He was being cared for by a brother who was only slightly older than he was. There were no other siblings. Their father had died two years earlier.

The patient was in a hospital bed located in the lower level family room in the home where an old grandfather clock sat, which had been lovingly cared for by the father prior to his death. It required frequent winding to work, and that hadn't happened since their father died. The patient's illness progressed, and he continued to decline steadily. He died in the presence of the social worker, the hospice nurse, and at least a dozen family friends. It was a tremendous loss for the older brother, and he was devastated.

Shortly after the funeral, the brother asked if he could meet with the social worker for lunch. When they got together, he shared a story that has stuck with the social worker for many years. Prior to his brother's death, the caregiver had asked his brother if he would send him a sign that he had made it to heaven and was reunited with their father. It happened that within 24 hours of losing his younger brother, a sign came. At 6:00 pm on the evening following the death, the older brother had gathered numerous friends in the family room where his brother had died the evening before. All were chatting and mourning together when suddenly the grandfather clock struck six times. This was a clock that had not been wound or chimed since the death of their father two years earlier.

For the surviving brother, this turned out to be the sign he had hoped for, that his brother and father were reunited in heaven. The clock did not strike again after that evening. This unexplained occurrence did more to comfort the older caregiving brother than anything else that might have happened. Moments like this can bring comfort to those who survive the loss of a loved one when they desperately want to know that their loved one is safely home. They are also comforting to those who work with the dying and remind us that as we stand at the bedside of the dying, we are standing on holy ground and in awe of the great mystery of life and what lies ahead.

(Social worker)

"Death ends a life, but it does not end a relationship..."
Robert Woodruff Anderson

Innocence and More Connections

Maureen was a patient who was in the last stages of a cancer diagnosis. She had a granddaughter who was only three years old and was diagnosed with leukemia and getting chemotherapy. The little girl, Sarah, was sitting at the end of her grandmother's bed in a chair that was high enough for her little legs to be sticking straight out from the seat of the chair. She was looking at grandma and appeared to be talking to her, but it seemed like she was really talking to someone else. She was asking questions, not directed to grandma, and she was getting answers from this "imaginary" person. She would answer, "OK," and the conversation seemed to continue. The hospice nurse said to the little girl, "who are you talking to?"

Sarah answered, "Nana's angel. You don't see Nana's angel?" The nurse answered, "No." This little girl was truly talking to someone because she'd make a statement, then she'd listen, and then she'd answer or say something, and then she'd stop and listen again. She wasn't just rambling on. The nurse told her that not all of us could see what special people could see. And that Sarah was a special person, a special little girl, and that was why she could see the angel. The nurse asked the little girl what "Nana's angel" was telling her. She said that "Nana's going to be

160

OK." Sarah said the angel was telling her that grandma was alright and she would not be here long but that it was OK because she was going to be OK. Nana was going to be fine and happy, and Nana's angels were going to take care of her. The angel was going to stay with her, and she was not leaving Nana's side. She said that when she had to go home, she would know Nana's angels were with her. In talking to the mother of this little girl, she shared that Sarah had been talking to Nana's angels for some time.

(Hospice nurse)

She's Over There

Hospice had been providing care for an elderly lady who had died. The hospice nurse was called at the time of death and was present with the family taking care of arrangements with the funeral home as the family was notifying other family members. The family had come, and all were gathered in the home. A little granddaughter who was two or three years old was also present with the family. The funeral home had been called and had arrived. When arrangements had been discussed, and it came time for the removal of the beloved grandmother, the funeral director lovingly placed the cot into the hearse. Everyone was standing together as they watched the hearse pull away from the home. But the little girl was standing and waving in the opposite direction from where the hearse was heading. A family member asked the little girl who she was waving at. She said, "Grandma, she's out there, right over there. And she's going up." When the family explained that grandma was in the hearse driving away and questioned her further, she said, "No, grandma's not in that car that left; she's right over there."

(Hospice nurse)

I Already Know

Audrey and Walter had one of those unique relationships that, despite appearances, was deeply affectionate and loving in a bumpy sort of way. Affection was shared through barbs, contradictions, and at times less than tasteful communication. They had shared many years together and found themselves living in an Assisted Living community. Audrey had been showing signs of dementia, and her personality was at times a demonstration of some decrease in respect, most likely attributed to dementia. She seemed to be losing some of her capacity to filter her comments. Dementia has a way of stripping people of many aspects of their dignity. She was a vocal lady, and no thought was left without expression, both good and bad. She was pleasant the majority of the time, but on occasion, the sharp side of her dementia personality would come through.

Evidence of Audrey's dementia was increasing, and it was determined she would benefit from placement in the nursing home, which was attached to the Assisted Living facility. Her loving husband, Walter, was no longer able to care for her in their apartment. She was struggling to get settled in her new environment, and as often happens with dementia patients, the change in environment and transition to unfamiliar surroundings seemed to be causing her additional distress. The change in environment had obviously affected Audrey as she could be found sitting in her Geri-chair in the hall at the nursing home or even in her room, calling out for her beloved "Waaal.....ter, Waaal....ter, Waaal....ter" repeatedly. She was unable to find comfort in this new environment and was lonely for her husband. Her condition continued to deteriorate slowly, and with continued decline and change in her physical and mental status, it was deemed she was appropriate for hospice care. She was admitted, and the staff kept Walter updated on her progress.

She was supported and was as comfortable as could be expected despite the loss of companionship of her dear husband. After a period of time with ongoing communication with Walter and attention to his status, it became apparent that he, too, might be appropriate for hospice with the health problems that plagued him. Sometimes it happens that one spouse is admitted, and not long after, the other one declines and then becomes appropriate as well.

Walter was consequently admitted to hospice, and sadly his condition started to deteriorate quite rapidly. His symptoms were increasing, and it was determined his symptoms would be best managed in the hospital setting. He was admitted to the hospital for care that required some hospital treatment methods. He continued to deteriorate rather quickly, and as family was updated, the out-of-town son was advised it would be most appropriate for him to come home sooner better than later, as Walter's trajectory of decline was increasing. The son made arrangements and was quickly on his way. He lived about five to six hours away, and it was getting on into the late evening hours. He would travel through the night to get to his father's bedside as quickly as possible. At this time, Audrey was unable to fully comprehend the seriousness of the nature of Walter's condition, even though she was told that Walter was not doing well and he was in the hospital.

Walter was starting to drift in and out of consciousness, and he was informed that his son was on his way, the distance he had to travel, and approximately how soon he would be arriving. Walter seemed to be changing more quickly and was getting closer to death. He was supported by hospice managing his symptoms and was told it was OK if he was struggling and unable to hold on until his son arrived. His son would be arriving by early morning, but Walter continued to change quickly and died during the night before the son was able to arrive at the hospital. Everyone was feeling bad at having to share the information about his death with Audrey. When she awoke the next morning, the staff at the nursing home went into her room to share the sad news that her dear Walter had died. To their surprise, Audrey interrupted their report by telling them she already knew Walter had died during the night. She was able to convey to them that she knew because he had come to her through the night and told her he couldn't hold on. The son arrived in the morning and was also astonished at the gift of insight his mom received from his dad at his passing.

Once again, we stand in awe at the marvelous unfolding of the incredible gifts that come to us as witnesses at a most beautiful time in life and in death.

(Hospice nurse)

A Man's Best Friend

Hospice was serving this elderly man. He was a quiet, gentle man and had a wonderful wife. He had a dog, and they were very close. As the man was confined to his bed, the dog was always on the bed, near the foot of the bed, to be close to his master. It was a small dog, and when it went outside and came back in, it always jumped right back up on the bed. It was always with this man, his constant companion. The dog never stood on the bed but just lay near his beloved master.

This gentleman was getting closer to death, and the hospice nurse was called and came to the house to assist the family. She was standing with the family at the bedside, and the wife decided to go into the kitchen to prepare some food for those present. The nurse stayed at the bedside. As the family gathered in the kitchen and with the nurse at his side, the man took his last deep breath and died peacefully. At the same time he took his last breath, the dog immediately stood up on the bed, looked up at the corner of the room, and began to howl. The nurse described it as an eerie, keening kind of sound. The beloved dog just kept it up. The nurse left the bedside and went out into the kitchen to let the family know the beloved man had died. The dog kept on howling. The family had attempted several times, yelling at the dog to stop, but it just kept on howling and keening. Then, all of a sudden, the dog stopped, put his head down, got down from the bed, and went out into another room. The family reports the dog never went back into that bedroom again.

Because of the close relationship the man had with his dog and the persistent howling following this man's death, the family was concerned the dog might not allow the funeral home to come and remove the body from the home. But once the dog left that room, it never again went back into that room. The dog had said its final goodbye to its master and never needed to go back into the bedroom again.

(Hospice nurse)

A Spiritual Themes
The Pretty Lady Who Came

I attended the wake for the young daughter of some old family friends. I was not aware of the specifics of the death other than knowing the deceased was forty-something and was leaving three young children. She had twins who were less than a year old and a little girl around three years of age.

I went to the visitation early on the day of the funeral and arrived early before the parents came. Alone in the funeral home, I found myself amazed by the number of memorial expressions that filled the rooms. There were flowers, trees, chimes, and statues filling two large rooms at the funeral home. There were at least a dozen or more statues of different size angels.

When the parents arrived, we hugged and walked toward the casket together. On the way, the mother told me of the experience she had from the day before when they first arrived at the funeral home. She and her husband were taking their three-year-old granddaughter to see her mother's body. They walked through the maze of memorials viewing statue after statue, floral arrangements, chimes, and much more, when the little girl suddenly tugged very firmly on her grandmother's hand until she stopped. They happened to be standing right in front of one of the many angel statues. The little girl stopped, looked at the arrangement, and said to her grandmother, "That's the pretty lady that came to our house last night to get mommy."

The innocence of this little child allowed her to see "God things" that adults often fail to allow our minds to comprehend. Knowing the little girl was comforted by seeing an image that reminded her of the pretty lady who came to get her mommy also became a comfort to a grieved mother. Hopefully, this little girl and her grandmother will both be comforted when remembering that this young mother is safe in the presence of a pretty lady forever.

(Hospice volunteer)

It's Beautiful

This gentleman I had been caring for was actively dying in his home. The family had surrounded him and were singing Christian songs and praying. I was off to the side, just being present and available if the family needed support, when he sat up in bed, opened his eyes, and said, "Loot at that! It's beautiful." When his daughter asked him what he was looking at, he said, "Heaven, it's beautiful!" Who could ask for a more precious moment?

(Hospice nurse)

A Journey of Forgiveness

As a hospice chaplain, one of the first patients I was blessed to serve was a gentleman I will call Mr. L. He was a Navy Veteran who enjoyed talking about his tour of duty in the Navy and his time spent on various aircraft carriers. He was very proud of his country but seemed to have one very big obstacle that turned the pride of his military service into an internal struggle he could not seem to overcome.

Whenever Mr. L would talk about his military service, he would quickly come to tears as he recounted the realization that he had "killed so many young men" as part of being a soldier for the United States of America. He understood and acknowledged why he had to do what he did as part of his military and patriotic duty, but he was hampered by the belief that God would not forgive him for such horrific actions, even if it was as a soldier trying to survive on the battlefield.

It took nearly a year of bi-monthly visits with Mr. L, and many tears shed between the two of us as I tried to help him make the spiritual journey that would include forgiveness within himself and the acceptance of forgiveness from God. Mr. L believed forgiveness could be possible from the God he knew, loved, and had faith in, but he struggled to find a way to embrace this thinking for himself.

And then, one day, as I walked into his room with his wife sitting beside him, I saw this huge grin on her face. She called me over to the bedside and said to me, "Donna, you did it! He told me today that because of the work you have done, because of the prayers that the two of you have shared, and because God has finally reached inside his heart, he knows and believes he will see the face of God and be forgiven of his sins. Donna, he has been saved anew, and he says it is because of you!" As I looked at Mr. L, I could see he was a new man. He had a glow of peace there aren't words to describe. I give such great thanks to God for allowing me to make this journey with Mr. L and his wife.

At that moment, the three of us prayed together as we had never prayed before. We thanked God for the gift of forgiveness and for the friendship we had between us. We thanked him for this journey that had provided Mr. L with the peace he needed to let go and die peacefully with a complete and humble heart and mind.

Mr. L. died three months after he received God's grace in his heart. His wife called me when he died and told me she believes God brought us together for a reason, and she will be eternally grateful for the care, support, and guidance provided to her and Mr. L. She shared that she and Mr. L saw me as one of the family and they would never forget me. I reflected the same sentiment about them back to her, and to this day, I have never forgotten them. His picture hangs on my office wall and reminds me daily how blessed I am to walk this hospice journey with patients and their families and all in the name of a loving and amazing God.

One of the hardest obstacles to peace at the end of life is the issue of forgiveness. Many people struggle not so much with forgiving others but with self-forgiveness. The end of life brings to the surface issues that may have been forgotten, denied, or hidden from our memory over the years. Helping people find peace and contentment in the life they have lived is a big part of making sure the journey each of them walks will bring them to the best place possible as they make their way from this world to the next.

Moments of forgiveness are a crucial part of the end of life work.

(Spiritual care coordinator)

Unexpected Blessings

Ronnie was a quiet little lady in her 80s and had lived a life that was not always easy. She was no stranger to abuse early on in life, with periods of the same kind of struggle throughout her life. Despite her history of hardship, Ronnie never spoke of any of her past history or felt sorry for herself. Rather, she tended to carry a sense of personal responsibility for what happened in her life. Her generational sense of personal accountability was not uncommon.

She came into our hospice program with an enlarging tumor growing out of the left side of her neck. We were naturally concerned about the potential for tumor growth and encroachment of the major vessels in her neck. She seemed unfazed by these potential concerns we had about her physical status. I visited Ronnie frequently and would always find her in her room at the nursing home where she resided. She was private and didn't particularly enjoy social activities. She was content in her little cocoon of a world in her room.

With time, Ronnie seemed to "open up" and trust our services and my visits. She was willing to share short conversations but never really revealed anything personal. I loved the visits and bringing a little sunshine with light conversation and soft humor to brighten her day. Visiting with her meant a lot to me. She was becoming more and more comfortable with the visits as the days and weeks rolled on. Her tumor continued to grow, and we monitored her diligently. She seemed to look forward to my visits.

On one particular visit, I remember sitting beside her on her bed, offering a little upbeat, lighthearted conversation after my clinical assessment. She proceeded to tell me that the priest from her home parish had visited the previous day, and she had received the Sacrament of the Anointing of the Sick. She was a little perplexed, though, noting that the priest had also blessed her hands, and she couldn't quite understand what that meant. Being of the same faith tradition as Ronnie and knowing that the Sacrament of the Sick included anointing of the hands, I was moved to explain that I thought it was the most beautiful thing to do for her. He was blessing her hands for all the work and efforts put forth in her lifetime through her hands. He was blessing all that those hands had accomplished in her life, many of which she may never have realized the importance of or how, through her hands, many people had been blessed. Inside, I hoped the words would be of some comfort to her.

A few moments passed, and she tenderly looked me in the eyes and said, "I don't think I've ever known anyone like you." All I could think to say was, "Well, that might be a good thing." She smiled broadly, and I could see in those eyes a deep, genuine affection she was offering with that statement as she shared an appreciation for the compassion and unconditional concern and support shown to her. I will never forget that moment of connection with this most amazing lady. I felt privileged to get to know her, even if only a little. That moment, she put an indelible impression on my heart. I know she carried a sense of guilt about many of the parts of her life, and I hope she was able to find some small sense of solace through that unusual blessing.

A few years after having cared for Ronnie, I was also able to care for a very beloved and well-respected track coach from the community who had been diagnosed with a brain tumor at a young age. As I journeyed with him and his family, I often thought how wonderful it would be to have someone bless this man's feet. Those feet and the heart they carried in his body had influenced and impacted many people through his efforts as a coach and running enthusiast.

The work of our hands, our feet, or any part of us that reaches out to help others is worthy of recognition and blessing as they have been the instrument of blessing to many through the years.

(Hospice nurse)

Peace in Prayer

Howard was in our hospice program, and we had been seeing him in Assisted Living. He needed to be moved to a "Memory Care Apartment" as his Alzheimer's disease was progressing. The hospice nurse and aide would visit several times a week, and he would relate the same stories at each visit about where he lived with his brothers and sisters across from the church. This seemed important to him. We came to realize he had lived a faith-filled life as he included this story each time we saw him.

Howard's journey seemed to be closing in on his final days, and his son had arrived to be with him. He seemed to be restless during this particular visit. The son was present, and a religious sister from his home parish had arrived. The restlessness seemed to continue. We decided that knowing his religious history, maybe he would be comforted if we prayed. So it was decided to say the "Our Father" as we gathered around his bed, and he could hear us in prayer. As we stood around the bed, praying this favorite prayer, Howard seemed to calm, and it was only moments later he took his last breath. This man of faith was able to find his way home as he was supported with the familiar prayer of his long life of faith. He was now home again with his God and his wife.

We get to witness many moments of inspiration as we

humbly journey with so many. Sometimes understanding the life they lived and what was important to them gives us clues to what will help them find their way home in a most peace-filled and perfect way.

(Hospice nurse and Hospice aide)

Recognizing Jesus

Joe's house was small and a little run-down looking. As I walked up to the door, I could see the upper hinge was coming off the door, and the screen had a few holes in it. I knocked on the door, and a young lady introducing herself as Tammy, Joe's caregiver, answered. I introduced myself as the hospice aide assigned to Joe's care. She directed me to the room where Joe slept and said she would run a few errands while I was there with Joe. I assured her I would be just fine.

Joe was resting in bed but awakened easily as I called his name. I introduced myself and told him why I was there. I said I was happy to help him with personal care, a shower, a shave, and maybe a clean shirt. I hoped Joe would agree that sometimes a warm shower is better than any medication. Joe was not very talkative. He was a quiet, gentle man with the softest blue eyes I have ever seen. I could tell we were going to need time and a couple more visits to build a rapport. Many times I have thought about how difficult this must be for my patients. Not only are they dealing with a stranger coming into their home, but also the acceptance of failing health and needing help with basic cares. I was perfectly fine with this introductory visit of talking and letting Joe get to know me. I also wanted to know more about Joe. I tried to throw in a little humor here and there, but it was clearly a one-sided conversation. Joe did not offer much to the conversation.

Joe's caregiver returned within an hour, and I thanked Joe for the opportunity to visit with him. I asked him if I could return later in the week, and at that time, he could decide if I could help him in any way. Joe nodded his head yes, but not with much enthusiasm.

Joe's health was declining a little more each time I saw him. He was getting weaker, and he wasn't eating or drinking much. Each visit was pretty much the same. I did most of the talking. Joe listened. He smiled occasionally. Gradually we got to know each other, and Joe accepted my help. I bathed him in bed for his comfort. All finished, I sat at his bedside. I took his hand in mine and told him how handsome he looked, being all cleaned up. I felt the gentle squeeze of his hand, and a little smile appeared on his face.

I have always believed that Jesus walks this earth. He takes the form of many human beings. We never know if, when, or where we will encounter him as we go about our busy, everyday life. He may be the person you held the door for or the person you let move ahead of you in traffic. He may be the crabby person waiting in line or the homeless man you bought that sandwich for.

As I left Joe's house that day, something occurred to me. I may have just given Jesus a bath.

(Hospice aide)

Pray for Me at the Hour of My Death

Marta was handicapped from birth. She was now in her 50s with the mental capacity of an eight or nine-year-old. She was a very spiritual woman who attended Mass at her local and nearby church every morning. She never missed Mass. She was very devoted to her faith and would pray two or three rosaries daily. She wasn't able to read and comprehend all that was in the Bible, but she knew her prayers, and she had a great devotion to the Blessed Mother Mary. She had lived in her parent's home until she was no longer able to care for herself.

She was admitted to the local nursing home as her health had been declining, and she was no longer able to care for herself with all her medical needs. As her health was declining, she appeared to be nearing death, and the nursing home staff noted she was becoming increasingly anxious. She had a sister and brother-in-law, and they wanted some help for her, but they did not know what to do for her. She had been fairly independent in life, and they hadn't been intimately involved in her care. With her increasing agitation and anxiety, they knew they needed some help for her. There seemed to be nothing that helped her restlessness, and she continued to be unable to settle down to a peaceful state.

A hospice nurse happened to be present in the facility

seeing other patients and knowing how much hospice can help with restlessness in the dying, the nursing home staff approached the hospice nurse and asked her for her help and what could be done to help this dear lady find some comfort and peace. Marta was not, unfortunately, in the hospice program, but the compassion and sensitivity of the hospice nurse drew her to the bedside to see if there was anything that could be done to allow this lady to be more comfortable and peaceful. The staff nurse and the hospice nurse could not allow her to continue in her state of distress that the family and staff were witnessing. Maybe she needed to be admitted to hospice for more support and comfort care.

The hospice nurse sat down at her bedside and took her hand in her own, and started to talk calmly to her. She was informed by staff and family about Marta's history and that she was a kind woman and a very faith-filled lady with a deep devotion to the Blessed Mother with years of devotion and prayers to Mary. Hearing this history of Marta and being of the same faith tradition, the hospice nurse started telling Marta that every time she had been praying the rosary and saying the Hail Mary that she had been praying for this very moment when she herself was at the hour of her own death. Every time she said, "Holy Mary, Mother of God, pray for me now and at the hour of my death", she was asking Mary to be here at this moment with her. The nurse continued to hold her hand and told Marta to keep holding on to the nurse's hand until Mary came and she could see her, and then Mary could take her hand, and she would guide her into the next life of eternal rest.

With continued reassurance from the nurse, Marta began to calm down slowly and became less restless and quite peaceful. She did not need any medication, just the reassurance that what she had prayed for all those years was now going to be given to her. The nurse assured her she would stay with her, and as any signs of restless agitation would surface, the nurse would again reassure her she would not leave her side until she was safely home. With all those rosaries she had said over the years, she would surely see the Blessed Mother.

Anytime the hospice nurse would try to loosen Marta's grip on her hand, Marta wouldn't let go. She would not even let go so the nurse could tell the sister what was happening or call the doctor. Reassured that the nurse was present and that Mary, the Blessed Mother, was coming to her was comforting beyond what any medication could possibly provide to this lady whose life was dedicated to her faith. Eventually, the nurse felt the loosening of Marta's grip on her hand, and Marta finally let go of the hospice nurse's hand. A beautiful smile had come over her face as she took her last breath. Marta had finally received the beautiful conclusion of her lifelong dedication to her faith and devotion to Mary. Mary had come to her at the hour of her death to finally take her home.

(Hospice nurse)

" It's All So Silly"

Jay and Mary had just "celebrated" their 17th wedding anniversary. He had been enduring a two-year battle with cancer, and it was obvious he was continuing to lose ground. They had three busy young children, and Mary had tried to maintain a sense of balance in their lives, caring for her dear husband and still attending to the active lives and activities of the children. She had worried many times about not being present with him at the time of his death. He had kindly refused much outside help and often told her, "I only need you." Their love grew much deeper during the time they navigated the many unknowns of a terminal illness. Jay had been able to cope with the terminal diagnosis by essentially living in denial. It was what worked for him as he proclaimed he was going to survive and no one was going to raise his children. He loved being a father more than anything in the world, and getting the diagnosis at a young age certainly altered his plans for life. Mary was very supportive of him in whatever way he needed throughout those months. They were trying to make the best of time out of the worst of time.

With the evidence he was declining, Mary had great concerns that if Jay died, he would not be happy if he were not with her and the children. She struggled to say the words "Thy will be done" from a favorite prayer, The Our Father. She found herself in church one Sunday morning, telling God that she just could not say those words with any truth or conviction. It was all weighing heavy on her heart, knowing that Jay seemed to be closing in on his final days, and he just did not want to die. Mary had always been the caregiver in their lives. Who would take care of him if he died? In a moment of inspiration while struggling in the church to pray, she thought that maybe if she could give him to Mary, the Blessed Mother, she might be able to find comfort in that. He needed someone to take care of him, and she felt if she could give him to Mary, that would help him and would ease her aching heart. It was all feeling too unbearable until she realized the Blessed Mother had also stood at the foot of the cross as she was witness to the torture and death of her beloved Son. Mary thought if the Blessed Virgin Mary could do it, then she herself must also find a way to do it with the grace that is always provided by our Loving Father in Heaven. She knew Jay had become accustomed to watching the rosary on TV each afternoon, and their faith, though challenged, did not waver. She had to find a way to trust her faith in God.

A few days following her profound spiritual insight at church, she found that around mid-afternoon, Jay seemed to be getting confused, and he shared with her that the ceiling seemed to be moving. Not completely aware of what was happening, she assured him it would be alright and the rosary he found comforting would soon be on TV. He then lifted his arm, and, making a circular motion with it, he proclaimed, "Mary, this is all so silly. 'In response, she asked, "What, Jay?" and again he responded, "All of this, it's all just so silly", again making the circular motion overhead with his hand. He was sitting in his recliner in their living room, and she started to become more concerned with each passing moment. She realized he was becoming less coherent, and she knelt down right in from of him in the recliner and took him in her arms. She was looking directly into his eyes when he seemed to be looking right through her, at something beyond her. He said, "Tell Dr. J this is 'wonderful'!" with an inflection in his voice she had never heard him use, even when referring to his most prized possession, an antique car. Not really understanding what was happening and knowing he had just eaten a small ice cream treat, she asked if he was referring to the ice cream. He was again staring right through her with an expression of amazement as he again said, "Yes, this is 'just wonderful'!" It was only moments later when she was holding him, and he began to sigh as if taking a last breath. She held him in her arms and said, "Come on, Jay, please just take one more last big breath for me." And he took that one last, long, deep breath, and it was his last. She then realized that the rosary they had been watching on TV had just finished, and in that instant, she knew without a doubt that Mary had come to take her beloved husband home with her.

Although distraught with the anguish of loss and sadness at the death of her beloved husband, Mary realized that through the eternal goodness and mercy of their Loving Father in heaven, Jay had been able to give her some reassurance in his final words of wisdom. Mary had always been the responsible one who tried to keep his lighthearted feet on the ground, and Jay was the happy-go-lucky guy that filled her life with love and humor. He was able to impart to her the wisdom that this life isn't what it's all about. As he said, this life is all "so silly". And we should not get caught up in it as our Loving Father in heaven has things much greater in store for us after we leave this life. She also knew that he would also be lovingly cared for as he was now with Mary, Our Blessed Mother. And he was able to help her realize that her concern for him being upset leaving her and the children wouldn't lie as traumatic on her heart because he knew there was something better waiting for all of them. He would be waiting for each of them one day in the next world. Her heart could be content knowing he was going where it was "wonderful, just wonderful."

There was no greater gift she could have received than those reassurances and the wisdom imparted to her by her beloved Jay. As his last words settled into her heart, she realized most profoundly that it is not in this world that we will realize the great reward God has in store for us, and He is always close by to share His grace and mercy as we struggle through the challenges we face in this lifetime.

There is a wise saying attributed to several sources. "On the day you were born, you cried, and the world rejoiced. May you live your life so that on the day you die, the world cries and you rejoice." That saying seemed to be more than appropriate for them.

Months later, as Mary was struggling to get ready for work one morning and feeling overwhelmed with the challenges of being a single parent, work demands, and finding her way through grief, she was taken aback when the lyrics of this song on the radio caught her attention. She felt without a doubt that her loving husband was sending her a message from above as she listened to these lyrics of the song.

Just Remember, I Love You

By Firefall

When it all goes crazy, and the thrill is gone,
The days get rainy and the nights get long
When you get that feelin' you were born to lose
Staring at your ceiling thinkin' of your blues
When there's so much trouble that you wanna cry
The world has crumbled and you don't know why
When your hopes are fading, and they can't be found
Dreams have left you waiting, friends have let you down

Just remember I love you, And it'll be alright.

Just remember, I love you More than I can say

Maybe then your blues will fade away
When you need a lover, and you're down so low
Ya start to wonder, but you never know
When it feels like sorrow is your only friend
Knowing that tomorrow you'll feel this way again
When the blues come callin' at the break of dawn
Rain keeps fallin', but the rainbow's gone
When you feel like crying, but the tears won't come
When your dreams are dyin', when you're on the run

Just remember I love you, And it'll be alright

Just remember, I love you More than I can say

Just remember I love you, And it'll be alright

It'll be alright. It'll be alright. It'll be alright...

Songwriter: Rick Roberts.

(Hospice nurse)

In the months and years that follow a deep loss, there are moments when newfound insights and growth can be found in the most unforeseen or unusual places or circumstances. This insight may come from any number of resources. It may be a song, a poem, an experience, or even the backstory contained in a movie.

In the movie "Good Will Hunting," a mathematical genius finds himself with what he believes is a sure understanding of all things in the world. He sees a wise but sad and hurting therapist. In one therapy session, this wise therapist challenges the young genius when he confronts him with the concept of what true love is. The wise therapist who has known deep loss confronts him with a startling new understanding of true love. He tells the young man true love is not what you read in poems or books, or sonnets. The therapist tells him he knows nothing of true emotional love until he has sat at the bedside for hours on end of someone who is truly beloved and knowing that visiting hours have no meaning for him. That true love often surfaces from the most difficult and even tragic moments in life when all else seems to fade away except for that which stands firm between two people against all odds. It is the deep moments of heartache and facing the insurmountable challenges in life where true love shows itself.

Surviving after deep loss brings many sad moments and challenges, but there can also be moments when the music of life reinforces our connection with those who have died. Here is another song that offers the hope of connection with those we have loved.

Unchained Melody
By The Righteous Brothers

Oh, my love, my darling, I've hungered for your touch
A long, lonely time, And time goes by so slowly,
And time can do so much Are you still mine?

I need your love I need your love
Godspeed your love to me
Lonely rivers flow To the sea, to the sea
To the open arms of the sea, yeah
Lonely rivers sigh "Wait for me, wait for me"
I'll be coming home, wait for me

Oh, my love, my darling, I've hungered, for your touch.
A long, lonely time And time goes by so slowly
And time can do so much Are you still mine?
I need your love, I need your love.
Godspeed your love to me

Songwriters: Joni Mitchell, Alex North, Hy Zaret.

Knowing that parting from a loved one may be the hardest thing we face in this lifetime, sometimes, if we look at it from a different perspective, we can see death not only as an "ending" but also as a "beginning".

194

I am Standing Upon the Seashore

By Henry Van Dyke, sometimes attributed to Victor Hugo

I am standing upon the seashore.
A ship at my side spreads her white
Sails to the morning breeze
And starts for the blue ocean.

She is an object of beauty and strength.
I stand and watch her until, at length,
She hangs like a speck of white cloud,
Just where the sea and sky come
To mingle with each other.

Then, someone at my side says: "There, she is gone !"
"Gone where ?"
Gone from my sight. That is all.

She is just as large in mast and hull
And spar as she was when she left my side,
And she is just as able to bear her
Load of living freight to her destined port.
Her diminished size is in me, not in her.

And just at the moment when someone
At my side says, "There, she is gone !"
There are other eyes watching her coming.
And other voices ready to take up the glad shout;
"Here she comes !"

And that is dying

The Caregiver's Prayer

Almighty God, Divine Healer of all,
Grant me, Your handmaiden,
Strength and courage in my calling,
Give to my heart, compassion, and understanding,
Give to my mind, knowledge, and wisdom,
Give to my hands, skill and endurance,
Especially, dear Lord,
Help me always to remember
the true purpose of my vocation

That of selfless service and dedication
To the weak and despairing of body and spirit,

~ In the Name of Jesus,

Amen

Part II: Health Care Choices

When someone receives the diagnosis of a terminal illness, everything changes. It is a turning point in life and a time when we start to question many things, especially those things that affect our hearts and souls. It is time to start looking at the future and how to make sure our wishes for what lies ahead will be heard, honored, and respected.

We are familiar with a "Last Will and Testament," by which we bequeath our valuables and direct the disposition of our belongings and possessions after death. But do we take the time, or are we concerned enough to make our wishes known for how we want to live out the remainder of our lives? It is as important to think about what kind of health care we want, the things we are willing to tolerate to have more time, and the things we are not willing to tolerate or suffer for the sake of more days. These choices for care will change with time, as we age, and begin to see the world from a different perspective. Our priorities and values change as time goes on and especially when our health changes.

One way to make sure our choices and wishes for our health care are known and honored is by having Advance Directives in place. Advance Directives include the "Living Will" and the "Durable Power of Attorney for Health Care" or "Medical Power of Attorney". There is also the POLST (Physician Order for Life Sustaining Treatment), which is actually a Physician's Order for care for persons with serious illnesses. These may vary from state to state, so it is important to speak to your healthcare provider and review each state's laws. The Durable Power of Attorney for Health Care designates a person who will speak for someone when unable to speak for themselves. It is also important to have a conversation with your DPOA-HC and family members, so everyone understands your wishes and agrees to honor them. Choices made in ICU or in stressful medical situations often do not reflect the patient's wishes, as those decisions are made during emotional stress. That is why it is important to make sure these documents are current and the appropriate people, health care providers, and hospitals have them in your file. A very useful and helpful guide is Dr. Angelo E. Volandes's book The Conversation, A Revolutionary Plan For End-Of-Life Care.

In making choices for health care, it is important to include any goals for care. Is the goal cure of an illness, avoidance of suffering, maintaining abilities and functions, having control over what happens to you and the quality of life, or maybe the opportunity to accomplish some personal goal? It is important to determine the priorities you now have for life based on your values, preferences, and your current clinical circumstances. It is a good time to review any personal goals such as trips, places to visit, special occasions or events to attend, or people to see or reconnect with. What do you cherish most in life? Is it people, connections, activities, abilities, hobbies, or things to accomplish? What in life is most important to you? It may be family, friends, religious connections or a host of other options. From where do you draw strength? Who or what is the source of your support? How do you want to spend the time available to you? In truth, these questions can be asked of us at any time in our lives to help center us and make the whole of our life the best it can be.

Another important aspect of looking at the care offered is to be sure all of your questions about your current health and the options for treatment are answered to your understanding and your current situation. You have a right to honest answers, always. With respect to treatment options or interventions, you may want to know all the choices available, not just the ones offered for treatment or cure. What might you expect from the illness (disease), and how will it affect you in the short term (6-12 months) or in the long term (3-5 years)? Are there any adverse or negative side effects with treatment? Is the goal cure, and is that even possible? If treatment will prolong your life, for how long? How might treatment change your life? What is the best that can be hoped for with treatments/interventions? How long might you live without treatment? Will the treatment create undesirable side effects that will impact your quality of life, and how? Are you making health care decisions based on what you personally want, or are you influenced by others? You need to understand all the options and the potential outcomes of those interventions to your satisfaction. Understanding these important factors is the only way to make sure you will be getting the care you truly want.

Health care today primarily focuses on the Traditional Medical Model of Care, which emphasizes the diagnosis of illness or disease and the subsequent diagnostic measures needed to determine appropriate interventions and treatment of that illness. The goal of care is curing the illness or disease. The focus and goal are disease identification with subsequent assessments, interventions, and treatments with restoration to optimum health.

Over the last half of the 20th century and ever since, healthcare has expanded into multiple specialty areas. There are specialists and sub-specialists in nearly every area of medicine:

Cardiologists, Pulmonologists, Neurologists, Oncologists, Rheumatologists, Gynecologists, Gastroenterologists, Dermatologists, Orthopedic specialists, Psychologists, Endocrinologists, Nephrologists, Otolaryngologists, Ophthalmologists.

And the list goes on and on. There are disease-specific specialists in basically anything that can go wrong with the body. Medicine, with these many specialty areas, is referred to as Multi-Disciplinary Care. Each group is an expert within that particular discipline. With the Traditional Medical Model of Care and this Multi-Disciplinary approach to care, no single discipline is assigned the care of the whole person. If a problem arises in one organ system, that specialty area addresses the issue. The disciplines work toward optimum health for that particular organ system.

Because of the multitude of advances in medical science and technology over the past 100-plus years and with the increasing knowledge within these specialty areas, people are living longer with chronic illness and disease. A recent report estimated that knowledge in medicine is doubling about every five years. Many of the options available today would have seemed like science fiction a couple of generations ago. The reality of modern medicine presents the potential problem of choosing too much or choosing too little of the available technology. How is someone to know what the best options for their health care are?

Having all the new technology and the many choices they offer presents a dilemma for an aging population. What is too much and what is too little when it comes to health care interventions? When thinking about health care, everyone should be thinking about what goals they might have for their health. What a person wants will change over time and will change when their health changes. Age, chronic illness, and disease will affect the goals for health care and the care desired. Whatever decisions are made, they should be put in writing in the form of Advance Directives or a Living Will. It is also important to identify and designate a Durable Power of Attorney for Health Care. Identifying the person most trusted to speak for someone when they are no longer able to effectively speak for themselves adds the assurance that a person's wishes will be honored. It is equally important to have a conversation with the DPOA-HC and, if possible close family members who will be standing and speaking on someone's behalf if they are no longer able to effectively communicate their wishes. The benefit of Advance Directives and having the conversation early assures your wishes will be known and also decreases the stress that comes with making a decision on someone else's behalf. Without advance information and specific directives, those making decisions on another's behalf generally feel guilty about whatever decision may be made. No one wants to leave a loved one with that feeling of uncertainty.

Health Care Choices can generally be grouped into three categories. They are:

• Aggressive Treatment - for longer life no matter what. I agree to CPR, Ventilator support, ICU, tubes, and any available technology and/or treatments to sustain life no matter what has to be endured. Quantity of life means more than Quality. This is an appropriate goal for every healthy individual. If nothing is in writing to direct the plan of care, the default in health care is always DO EVERYTHING.

• Limited but Quality Care - including hospitalization, IV medications but maybe no Intensive Care. Care would include treatments and interventions to manage symptoms and provide comfort but nothing aggressive that would impact the quality of life. It would include a desire for as much quality time as possible with a minimum of suffering. This would be a good time for discussion about the benefits and/or burdens of particular interventions, treatments, or even hospitalization. It should also include discussion of the potential outcome and consequences of treatment choices. It would be an appropriate time for a conversation about the benefits of Palliative Care with a better understanding of what CPR and resuscitation would mean and what the potential outcome of these interventions might look like for someone who may already have compromised health. Understanding what these interventions look like and the realistic expectations and outcomes from the effects of CPR or other interventions can have a profound impact on the decision to choose or forgo treatment. Persons with chronic illness or long-term disease states might benefit from Palliative Care at this time.

• Quality Comfort Care - care would assure a life of quality and symptom relief with the option of deciding on the benefit and/or burden of choosing to go to the hospital or Emergency Room to receive care and treatment. With this care, there would be an understanding that any interventions or treatments may not prolong life but would provide quality and comfort in the days ahead for someone. Many times when people are admitted to hospice, they verbalize they are tired of the repeated hospitalizations, doctor visits, repeated interventions, treatments, and the poking and prodding that comes with it. This may be the time when a person might choose to enjoy the remainder of the time available to them rather than undergo burdensome treatments. It would be an appropriate time to review goals for care and have a conversation about Palliative Care and, if appropriate, Hospice Care.

All too often in the current healthcare environment, when the probability of cure or improvement seems remote, palliative care or hospice care is not offered until it's almost too late. The benefit of early referral to hospice can make a big difference for not only the patient but also the family. These conversations about healthcare choices always seem too early until it's too late.

Sadly, there is often a gap between what EOL (End of

Life) care a person wants and what one gets. Having Advance Directives in place and a conversation with family or those closest to the patient are the best methods for assuring someone's wishes are known and will be honored. These conversations should occur before someone is in crisis or is in ICU. Earlier conversations that can be had around the kitchen table without stressful emotions allow for decisions that are based on a person's personal values and true wishes. Decisions made during a crisis or when someone is in the hospital or ICU are often impacted by emotions and are greatly influenced by those present at the bedside without regard to what the patient might want. Having the conversation sooner is always better than later. Because we can do something in medicine doesn't necessarily mean we should do it. There is a bigger picture to consider, and the patient is the most important person in that bigger picture.

In the film, Consider the Conversation, Dr. Ira Byock states: "As we are born and as we die, we'll be physically dependent on others...at both poles of human life, caring for one another is what we do...being physically dependent on others at the end of life doesn't make one undignified, it simply makes one human."

We don't consider the absolute physical dependence and vulnerability and even incontinence of infants and toddlers as being anything abnormal or undignified. Yet at the end of life, we're supposedly undignified if we become physically dependent on others. We are connected at both poles of human life. Caring for one another is what we do. It is part of our very humanity. It is hardwired within us.

Once a man, twice a child. We start out in life as an infant, a child in a state of dependency. We grow into adulthood, and then as we age and lose physical and cognitive abilities, many times we return to a state of dependency and may again need some of the assistance in life as when we were children. A return to dependency does not need to include loss of dignity.

When asked about some of the priorities people have when facing a terminal illness, most want to avoid suffering, have family near, maintain their mental abilities, and do not want to be a burden to others. Many people get lost in uncertainty when surrounded by medical experts and life-extending technology. If we want to do everything for our loved ones, we must not be afraid to look at the picture of their life holistically, not just the physical symptoms. This does not mean we ignore physical symptoms, but in a broader sense, we take into consideration all aspects of life. The social, emotional, and spiritual aspects of their life are as important as the physical.

Another aspect of life that concerns most people who are facing a limited number of days is whether or not their life had has had meaning. At turning points in life, many ask questions that speak to the heart and soul. People wonder, "Have I fulfilled my purpose in life"? Will I be remembered, and if so, what kind of legacy will I pass along to those who survive me? We all want to know we have lived for something more meaningful and a purpose greater than ourselves.

An ancient tradition of passing on personal values, beliefs, advice for future generations, and even blessings is called an "Ethical Will." The Ethical Will is a way to look back at the story of our lives and examine the values and principles that have helped to form us into the person we have become. It is an opportunity to share and reflect on our life experiences and remember those moments that have influenced us as human beings. It is an opportunity to remember the many gifts of heart, mind, and soul we have brought to this world through our living. Putting these reflections in writing in the form of an Ethical Will may just be the most valuable possession we can leave for our loved ones, especially the younger generations that follow us and who, at the current time, may have little or no interest in such things. I remember when my dear dad died, I wondered if he had always been the great man he was when we honored him at death. I wish so many times I had known more about him and that I would have had the foresight to ask more questions. It wasn't until later in life I realized how much more I wanted to know about him. Little do we realize that when we stand at the graveside and say goodbye to a loved one, that we are also saying goodbye to their story and so much history. We may not only be burying our loved ones but may also be burying a library of information and a wealth of knowledge. If our living loved ones want to add to the legacy they leave for survivors, one of the best ways is by writing an ethical will.

The following websites are good links to writing an ethical will:

https://www.everplans.com/articles/how-to-write-an-ethical-will

https://cdn.sanity.io/files/zzw4zduo/production/498f796abb5578d66c785b541c18f94a908dce6a.pdf

How Hospice Care is Different

People often wonder what is so different about hospice care. Obviously, if we are talking about hospice, there is evidence that the end of life is within the foreseeable future for someone. To better understand how hospice care is different, we need to look at the Hospice Model of Care for patients and contrast it with the Traditional Medical Model of Care.

The Hospice Model of Care is different from the current Traditional Medical Model of Care in that the Hospice Model of Care is about shifting the focus from fixing and curing the illness or disease to providing comfort and managing symptoms. It is not less care but more focused care. Instead of the diagnosis or illness being the primary focus for care, the focus is now on the patient, their comfort, and quality of life. The care is not driven by a diagnosis or treatment but by respect for the patient's comfort, wishes, and desires for care. Hospice Care is the most patient-centered model of care available. The patient and their comfort and quality of life become the focus of care. Everything about the patient is important. In this holistic approach, the emotional, psychosocial, intellectual, and spiritual aspects of life are as important as the physical well-being of the person. It is the most holistic approach to care available. If it matters to the person/patient, it matters.

Hospice is health care that specializes in caring for

persons who are dealing with a terminal diagnosis. It is the specialty area of medicine that deals with the end of life, dying, and death. It is specialty care that focuses on caring for those facing a life-limiting illness or disease. We may be unable to change the destination, but there is a great ability to affect the quality of the journey and relieve the suffering and distress during this part of the journey. Even though the care is for people who are in the last stages of life, the focus is not on dying and death. The focus is on helping people to have a quality of life and comfort as they live out the days they have available. Hospice is about living life to the fullest to the very end, not dying and death. It is about life. The focus is not on the endpoint, death, but on the journey and making the days ahead meaningful and filled with as much comfort and quality as possible. Hospice provides expertise in symptom control and pain management and provides the best quality time possible while supporting the patient and their family.

Hospice Care is comfort care without seeking aggressive or curative treatment for a disease or illness. Life expectancy for the illness or disease, if it were to progress along its "natural course," would be anticipated to be six months or less. The focus is not on curing the illness. With all the advances in science and technology, we can't always fix or cure what happens to go wrong with our bodies. Care is focused on relieving symptoms and optimizing patient comfort. It is not about giving up hope which is a common misunderstanding about hospice. Hospice does not take hope away from anyone. What someone hopes for may change over time, but there is always hope. Hospice care can neither hasten death nor prolong life beyond its natural course. It is about accompanying the person on their journey to the end of life and providing comfort, symptom management, information, education, and support to assure the best quality of life possible.

With modern medicine, people are living longer with chronic illnesses. With Palliative care, the prognosis can be greater than six months, even years, and the person can continue to seek aggressive or curative treatments. Hospice Care always includes Palliative Care, but Palliative Care is not always Hospice Care because of the prognosis and approach to care. The goal/benefit of both Palliative and Hospice care are the same: to improve the quality of life for both the patient and the family, to relieve and prevent suffering, to clarify and align medical goals and avoid repeat unwanted hospitalizations and ER visits. Both strive to promote the best quality of life possible as defined by the patient and family. Both offer comfort, dignity, and choice while providing patients with relief from the symptoms, pain, physical stress, and mental stress of a serious illness, whatever the diagnosis. It is care and treatments based on comfort, not cure of the underlying cause. The focus is on the management of any symptoms causing distress to the patient.

Hospice is all about compassion. It is about giving the person a voice. It is about honoring and respecting the person for who they are, where they've been, and their life story, and providing the comfort and dignity every human being deserves. It is about honoring and respecting each individual and their family system not only as unique but as worthy of the best care possible. It concentrates on care, not cure. It is not about changing someone or forcing anyone to do anything. It is not less care, but the more focused and best care.

It is not the goal of hospice to tell anyone what's best for them. Hospice affirms life and recognizes that death is a part of the process of living, just like birth is a part of the process of life. Hospice has no desire or ability to shorten or lengthen the number of days a person has available to them. Hospice offers options for care and management of symptoms distressing to the patient, and it is ultimately the person who decides what they choose for their comfort

The Hospice movement has done something dramatic to medicine in putting the patient back at the center of care, regarding them as a whole person as opposed to a disease entity. The person has a disease, and it is not that the disease has the person. In our technical, highly advanced medical environment, dying and death are frequently considered "a failure". Physicians are trained to cure, fix, and heal, to make better. Sadly, death is too often viewed as a failure to cure on the part of the doctor and even the patient. Too often, we hear that "the patient failed treatment". The patient doesn't fail the treatment; the treatment fails the patient. We must avoid putting the onus of failure on anyone, doctor or patient. This attitude of failure is oppositional to the idea that dying and death are simply another stage in the life cycle. There can be many accomplishments during the final stage of life. Dying and death can be essential to human development. They help us to live fully and become fully human right up to the very last moment of life.

For that to happen, technology and all health care must be infused with compassion and benevolence. Life is not just a matter of length but one of depth and quality as well. Controlling pain and other distressing symptoms in terminal patients is essential to allow their full potential to be lived out in the moral, spiritual, and ethical dimensions of their life.

Health care has a noble path to curing disease, but there doesn't seem to be the same noble path to dying. Dying is seen as failing. We have a heroic narrative for fighting together to cure illness and disease, but there isn't such a heroic narrative for letting go and dying.

Ira Byock: "You know, the best doctor in the world has never succeeded in making anyone immortal."

The holistic approach of hospice care focuses on the social, emotional, intellectual, and spiritual aspects of the patient as well as their physical comfort.

Sometimes treatment options or interventions offered actually bring more distress and suffering than a patient really wants to tolerate. Patients have a right, and healthcare providers have a responsibility to make sure the person fully understands all the options available to them and the consequences or potential outcomes of those choices. When someone fully understands all the choices and consequences of those choices, they are more fully able to make decisions that are in their best interest and that align with their health care goals.

It is not uncommon that patients and their families use denial to find ways to survive a terminal illness. Living in denial provides protection from the reality of what is happening. It becomes a powerful defense mechanism, and it is not anyone's job to tell the patient how to cope. No one should ever take away any hope of recovery, even if it seems remote and impossible. Denial becomes the lifeline that allows some patients to endure and get through each day. Eventually, patients may come to realize the reality of their situation and, in their own way, cope with the truth of what lies ahead. They may or may not express this understanding, and if they are unable to express it, that is OK. It is not appropriate or helpful to tell anyone how to cope or to take away any shred of hope there might be. No one has that right over any person.

Honoring and respecting how someone chooses to cope with their illness and bring their life to a close at death is part of the innate dignity afforded to every person who enters hospice care. Meeting them where they are on their journey without an agenda, expectation, or judgment of them offers the greatest dignity and honors them through whatever choices they make in their final days. It is the best way to offer the respect that each person deserves in this life. Every human being has a right to a self-determined life closure, bringing their life journey to its conclusion on their own terms.

It is sad that the importance of honoring and respecting the dignity of every individual's life oftentimes isn't recognized or regarded as important until that person is facing the end of life. How different the world would be if we were to treat each other throughout life with the concern, admiration, and respect offered through hospice care at the end of life.

Part III: What Does Dying Look Like?

The movies and TV do not give us a realistic picture of what to expect. Dying is simply the shutting down of the body's physical, sensory, and mental functions. It is not just a biological affair but a human one. It is a very personal time in anyone's life. Despite the multitude of advancements in medical technology and all the treatments and interventions at our disposal, each of us will face death someday. There isn't always a treatment or intervention, fix or cure for everything. Any technology offered throughout life and especially at the end of life, must be infused with compassion and kindness to have the best effect and for life to have a peaceful and grace-filled conclusion. These qualities are necessary for patients to feel respected and to eventually bring their life to a dignified conclusion.

There is no better classroom about the bedrock truth of life than the deathbed. The truth is that we are all only here for a short time. In life, we often lose perspective about what is important. At the deathbed, we find that what truly is most important is love, compassion, and the most basic of human connections, our kinship with others. There is no map for the territory of dying. At the bedside of the dying, we find that it is the simple things that matter most. Presence and silence speak volumes to the dying person.

They say you are important, you matter, and you are worth my time right now, without interruption or distraction. Journeying with the dying is humbling and grace-filled. Each death is as unique as the birth and life of the person who lived it.

In Joyce Rupp's book Boundless Compassion, we are told that "compassion asks us to go where it hurts, to enter places of pain, to share in brokenness, fear, confusion, and anguish." Compassion challenges us to cry out with those in misery, to mourn with those who are lonely, and to weep with those in tears. It requires us to be weak with the weak, vulnerable with the vulnerable, and powerless with the powerless."

In general, dying is the gentle retreating back into a vulnerable state like we experienced when we were infants. There is increasing weakness and decreased ability to perform personal cares and other usual daily activities. There is increased difficulty with ambulation as the body slows down and functional capacity decreases. Patients become weaker, more sedentary, and somnolent (sleepy, drowsy, tired) as their engagement in life and their environment decreases.

The decline in a person's status at the end of life is typically linear unless there is an acute event. This trajectory of decline can be medical, measured by labs, xrays, scans, etc. There can also be evidence of functional change. There are certain signs and signals that tell us the organs are in the process of shutting down. Changes occur in each organ system as the body begins to shut down. It does not seem to matter the diagnosis or illness that is the cause or source of the dying. The process tends to be familiar and similar no matter the reason for the dying. Unless it is an acute event or one that occurs from a tragic event, there are many similarities seen during the dying process.

Just like the body must go through certain stages to prepare to be born, it must also go through certain stages to shut down and die. The trajectory of decline can be noticeable changes in a person's status, clinical or functional, as measured from a year ago, six months ago, one month ago, or even a week or days ago. The shorter amount of time within which the change is noted indicates how rapid the decline in status is occurring, and the trajectory (typically linear) becomes steeper.

The first "organ system" where changes are typically noted is the digestive system. Other organ systems follow. There may be changes in conscious awareness and increasing changes in functional capabilities. The heart and lungs typically "shut down" last. Not everyone experiences all of the symptoms, but there are many common ones. It's important to note these physical changes do not happen in a specific order, and not everyone experiences all of them. Each person is unique in how they enter this world, and they are also unique in how they find their way to the next world. In his book Visions, Trips, and Crowded Rooms, David Kessler explains that "Deaths and births are like snowflakes-each one is unique and very similar." No two are alike, but there are great similarities.

The body has a natural wisdom built into it to protect itself and promote comfort. One of several reasons people will be more comfortable is because of hormones called endorphins. These are chemicals produced naturally by the nervous system to cope with pain or stress. They are often referred to as the brain's "feel-good" chemicals because they act as pain relievers and happiness boosters. They are the body's natural painkillers and, when released, will promote a sense of well-being and comfort. They are released from the pituitary gland in the brain and activate the body's opiate receptors to reduce the perception of pain, causing an analgesic effect. Endorphins trigger a positive feeling in the body, similar to that of morphine and codeine.

A Plan of Care for End of Life

A typical Plan of Care for an actively dying person addresses every aspect of their being. From a clinical perspective, there is a more liberal approach to developing a Plan of Care for someone whose life expectancy is shortened, and the finish line is in the foreseeable future. This is in contrast to someone receiving healthcare according to the Traditional Medical Model of Care.

For example, with cardiac or respiratory patients, fluid restrictions are less strict and more liberal for a dying person. Patients are encouraged to eat and drink as they desire and as they feel comfortable. There is also less concern for cholesterol or blood sugar levels. To avoid low blood sugars, insulin doses are typically decreased and often discontinued. Unless blood sugars are consistently>500, the adverse effects and damage of high blood sugars are minimal in the long run. Patients are encouraged to find joy in eating foods that are pleasurable to them, no matter the potential long-term adverse effects that were previously a concern. Most persons facing the end of life are not eating and taking in calories like a healthy person. Comfort trumps the traditional medical approach. Symptom management and comfort are priorities.

Food, Fluids, Nutrition, Appetite Changes, Difficulty Swallowing, and Dry Mouth

Food is symbolic of love and nurturing. The needs of the body and its ability to process and utilize food changes in the final months of life. As the body begins to shut down, it loses its ability to process food and fluids. There is a decreased need for food, fluids, and nutrition in general. The person may be more comfortable when not eating as the feel-good hormones are activated. With the decreased need for nutrition in general, the person begins to lose interest in eating or drinking and will even lose the sensation of being thirsty. With the organ systems slowing, the body naturally knows it doesn't need the same amount of calories as it has in the past. Encouraging intake at this time might even cause discomfort and distress for the person. Medications, the disease itself, food odors, or even tumor growth may become a source of nausea. Unlike a healthy person, a person at the end of life does not experience hunger or thirst the way a healthy person does.

Loss of appetite and thirst is a natural process by which the body begins to prepare itself for death. Clear signs of the GI system slowing down may include the patient taking longer and longer to finish a meal. They may clamp their lips shut or push away the hand that is feeding them, or even turn their head away when food is offered. They may desire a specific food, then only take a bite. Cold food can sometimes be more palatable. Narcotics which help with pain management and shortness of breath, can slow the bowels and lead to symptoms of constipation, bloating, or nausea. The desire for food and intake will continue to decrease, and they may eventually refuse to eat entirely.

Natural dehydration promotes the release of endorphins which promote increased comfort and a calming effect, decreasing pain and anxiety. If food or fluids are given artificially near the end of life, they may actually cause increased discomfort. Natural dehydration results in less chance of nausea and vomiting, swelling, and lung congestion. Excess IV fluids at the end of life can cause complications such as edema (swelling within the tissues), as well as "fluid overload". Fluid overload (having too much fluid in the tissues of the body) can cause many distressing symptoms.

Difficulty swallowing is a common symptom that occurs in the majority of patients with a life-limiting illness. Swallowing disorders are part of the natural process at the end of life. Muscle wasting, slowing of natural reflexes, cachexia (weakness and wasting of the body due to severe chronic illness), and physical weakness affect the coordination and muscle strength needed for swallowing. Dysphagia (difficulty or discomfort in swallowing) is a major predisposing condition for aspiration (inhaling food, liquid, or other substance into the lungs) or choking.

All organ systems are slowing down in preparation for death, and *people do not die because they are not eating. They are not eating because they are dying.* That is another misunderstanding about the end of life. It is commonly feared that a loved one will "starve to death" or become dehydrated and suffer. In fact, the opposite is true. Adequate end-of-life nutrition is important. However, a person with a life-limiting illness in the later stages of life may experience physical symptoms that cause more discomfort or complications if forced to eat or drink when they do not feel the need to do so. In truth, if they are hungry or thirsty, they will indicate that need. Offering but not forcing is important to ensure their best comfort.

Care Includes: First and foremost; it is important to honor the patient's requests/desires. Allow the patient to determine what, how much, and how often they choose to eat or drink. Food and fluids should neither be actively forced nor actively withheld. A patient's body will tell them what they need and when they need it. Allow the patient to decide if or what they want to eat or drink with care for protection from aspiration.

Having the patient in an upright position with chin parallel to the floor is helpful. Tucking the chin down when swallowing liquids is also beneficial. Making sure the

223

person swallows before giving the next sip or even double swallowing, can help. Massaging the cheek to propel food toward the throat and limiting portions to ½ to 1 tsp. servings at a time reduces the risk for choking or aspiration. Alternate solids and liquids and have the person remain upright for 30 minutes after eating. All of these suggestions are easily implemented and are greatly beneficial to protect the person from choking or aspiration.

The person's diet for food and fluids can be downgraded as needed from regular consistency to ground, mechanical soft, soft, and eventually to full liquid. It is especially important to consider patient preference and use whatever measures are needed in an attempt to maintain nutrition but also to safeguard against aspiration. Eventually, as the patient enters into the active dying phase, it is appropriate to only offer food and fluids if awake and alert.

Drinking from straws is strongly discouraged due to the risk of aspiration. Allowing only drops of a desired liquid from a straw with great caution may be offered. Small amounts of ice chips or a Popsicle may be welcome. Distaste for thickened liquids can increase the risk of dehydration if the patient doesn't care for the taste or texture of the thickened liquids. Patients should be fully informed of the consequences and risks if choosing to continue on thin liquids when it is apparent they are having difficulty with swallowing. Check with your hospice care team for appropriate suggestions.

Oral cares and oral hygiene are important and provide an element of comfort that is often overlooked. Brushing the teeth should be continued as the patient tolerates it. Care includes keeping the mouth moist, clean, and fresh for comfort. Moisten the mouth with oral swabs with care to remove excess liquid from the swab when there is an increased risk for aspiration. Swabs can be soaked in water or mouthwash, or if there is a desire for a specific liquid, that can also be offered by swab. Swabbing the mouth to clear it of secretions before administering any liquid medication promotes better absorption of the medicine. DO NOT swab the mouth following the administration of sublingual (under the tongue) liquid medications, as the swab will absorb the medication and decrease the amount of medicine the patient receives. Applying lip balm frequently can prevent cracking from dryness. Keeping the head of the bed slightly elevated during any intake will help to decrease complications associated with eating.

With decreased intake, bowel movements may decrease, but it is still important to monitor the frequency and consistency of stool and use stool softeners or laxatives as needed to keep the bowels from becoming sluggish. The hospice care team is always available for information and a supportive understanding of the best practices for any concerns relating to nutrition and the GI system.

Skin Changes - Circulation – Fever - Repositioning

The skin is the body's largest organ and, like any other organ, is subject to a loss of integrity. Circulation slows as body systems slow. Physiologic changes that occur as a result of the dying process may affect the skin and soft tissues and manifest as skin coolness, mottling (blotchy, red-purplish marbling of the skin, especially the extremities), and changes in skin turgor, or integrity. These skin changes are a reflection of decreased nutrition and circulation, resulting in reduced soft tissue perfusion, decreased tolerance to external insults, and impaired removal of metabolic wastes. There is an increased risk of injury due to both internal and external insults.

With decreased nutrition available, skin health changes and breakdown can occur. There is potential for rapid skin compromise. Minor insults can lead to major complications such as skin tears, pressure ulcers, hemorrhage, gangrene, and infection. Coldness in the limbs might be noted in the person's hands, arms, feet, and legs and are evidence that skin integrity is changing as blood circulation slows. As the body systems slow, blood may coagulate or pool, particularly at the base of the spine, with patches that look like dark purple bruising.

Care Includes: Cover to comfort, using lighter covers or sheets rather than heavy blankets. Use fans or open windows for air circulation. The body's thermostat center in the brain is less effective in regulating body temperature. A fever is NOT always an indication of infection. Tylenol or fever-reducing medications are not typically helpful. A cool cloth on the forehead can be comforting if desired. Positioning is important. Pressure or shearing (peeling, pulling, or wearing off), skin breakdown is secondary to the primary causative factor, which is skin organ failure. An air mattress or alternating pressure mattress can help to reduce pressure over bony areas. Frequent turning will help to decrease the incidence of skin breakdown and wound formation, especially over bony prominences. Turning from side to side, onto the back with pillow support behind the back or under or between the knees to maintain natural and comfortable body alignment is important. Placing pillows for support under the ankles to "float" the heels and feet helps to prevent pressure sores. Family may decline turning, thinking it may cause discomfort, but it is still important to inspect the skin for any rapid change or skin compromise. Bony prominences are most at risk. With any turning, inspect the skin for any indications of redness, compromise, or skin breakdown. If turning is not happening, it is still important to do a skin assessment for any changes, especially over those areas where bones are closest to the skin. Skin breakdown can occur suddenly and rapidly, which is why it is important to inspect the skin frequently.

Withdrawal - Change in Level of Consciousness – Neurologic Changes - Disorientation - Activity - Terminal Restlessness

Withdrawal can be the beginning of letting go. People who were always interested in their favorite activities, such as sports, may no longer worry or be concerned about their favorite team. Interest in the outside world decreases. There is less focus and less energy on the world around them, and they may appear to lose interest in their surroundings, favorite pastimes, and even visitors. It is not unusual for people to doze off during conversations. Communication becomes harder and requires more energy than it did previously. It's important to realize this is not a rejection of loved ones or visitors but a withdrawal from life in general. It takes a lot of energy to follow conversations, speak, and track what is going on in the immediate environment. As with everything else, their ability and desire for engagement in the greater world are decreasing. Their world begins to shrink. Imagine interest shrinking from the global stage of events and then just interest in what's happening nationally. Soon interest is limited to only what is happening statewide, then in their town, their street, only their house, their room, chair, or bed. It is a natural and progressive retreating from life and is not a reflection of rejection.

228

It is like the reversal of when we are born. We start out helpless with every need and care provided. An infant learns to roll over, crawl, walk, and run. Their encounter in the world continues to increase as a child enters school and creates friendships beyond the family. In high school, their world increases even more with new friends, jobs, and coworkers, and after graduation, their world expands even further. Life continues to keep growing broader and bigger. With aging and especially the end of life, there is a reversal and decreasing engagement in the greater world. Unless there is sudden death, the process of dying then is the gentle retreating back into a vulnerable state like we experienced when we were infants.

When the finish line is in the foreseeable future, there is increasing weakness in general and increased difficulty with ambulation. The person becomes less able to do personal cares, becomes more sedentary, and eventually becomes chair or bed-bound. There is great variance in the time within which these changes may occur. Every person's birth, life, and dying are unique to them. There are similarities, but uniqueness still exists for each person as they progress toward the end of life. With increased weakness, there can be more somnolence with less frequent periods of being fully awake and alert. This can partly be related to decreased oxygen to the brain and part of the natural progression of the body systems slowing down.

There is often increasing amounts of time dozing or sleeping, and they may eventually become difficult to arouse at times. The body's metabolism is changing, and the decrease in circulation and oxygen to the brain is a normal part of the process. In the last few days of life, people often drift in and out of consciousness. Eventually, they may appear to be unresponsive or in a coma-like state.

If the mind is distressed, the body typically follows the mind. Sometimes issues can be distressing to the patient and cause agitation or anxiety. They may be experiencing something referred to as Terminal Restlessness. Observable manifestations may be increased, non-purposeful activity, inability to relax, confusion, disorientation, sleep disturbance, impairment of judgment, or escalating anxiety. Activity or distraction does not seem to satisfy the person. There may be picking at the bed linens, or they may desire to get up from bed and sit in a chair and then almost immediately desire to move to another position or go back to the bed or chair. Whatever is done to satisfy a spoken need does not bring peace and satisfaction to the person. The mind is like a gerbil on the wheel going round and round. The mind is racing, and the body follows the mind with non-satisfying activity.

Identifying the source can be a challenge. The anxiety can be related to the person's fear of death or the dying process. There may be spoken or unspoken regrets or unmet spiritual needs. Sometimes unfinished business can include a person's need for the resolution of conflicts, reconciliation with another person, or identification of fears or disappointments. There can be many different reasons for the distress. The hospice team is trained to help identify the source if possible and should be made aware of any noted distress or restlessness. Medications can be helpful but may not always provide relief depending on what the issues are and how important they are to the patient.

Care Includes: Continue talking to your loved one and treat them as you normally would. They are still alive and present until their last breath despite their decreasing ability to engage with you. Use touch as you ordinarily would for their comfort. Maintaining a physical presence and touching the person gently without expecting anything from them provides the reassurance that they will not be abandoned during this phase of their life. Identify yourself by name whenever entering their presence, even if they are unresponsive. Do not challenge them to identify who you are. That takes energy on their part. Speak softly but calmly, clearly, directly, and as naturally as you would normally do. Explain any activities that might be happening or cares that might be anticipated. Hand-holding, quiet music, or reading softly may be calming if that has been something that was enjoyed in the past. It is good to keep conversations short. If you know they might be interested in something happening with family, friends, or in the community, share that information without expecting a response or interaction about it. They may be able to enjoy friendly conversation among those present as they listen to stories about the past or memories that have been particularly important throughout their lifetime. Maintaining a calm, quiet environment is much better than great excitement and noisy activity.

Reminiscing can be a beautiful way to honor them as those present remember contributions the person may have brought to life. Spending time with them when they are more alert can be beneficial. Sit with them, hold their hand, or provide any comforting measures you know they might appreciate. Do not shake them or speak loudly. Try to keep the environment calm and decrease the busyness of what's happening around them. Do not talk about them as if they are not present. Always assume they can hear you. We believe that hearing is the last sense to leave the body. It provides honor and dignity to treat them as fully alive until the very last breath.

For any restless activity, it is best to engage the hospice team to identify the source. Depending on the cause of the restless activity, measures can be taken to address the issue(s) and find the best possible resolution(s). It is important not to challenge or diminish the individual about their behavior or do anything that will increase the distress the patient may be feeling. Engage the hospice team to help identify the source and resolve the distress.

Confusion - Vision-Like Experiences - Symbolic Speech and Gestures.

The person may seem to be confused about time and place or unable to recognize or identify people in their presence, including family or close friends. They may appear to be talking to someone you cannot see or loved ones who have already died. They may talk of traveling, leaving, and packing, going on a trip, going home, or talking to unseen people as if they are present with them. These are not uncommon in the transition from life to death. Whatever they say may carry an importance. When they speak, we listen. They may be giving us clues about what is happening with them as they are transitioning from this world to the next. There may be some unfinished business they need to address. If there are issues that need to be resolved, it is important to determine what those might be and address them in whatever way possible to resolve any conflict that might interfere with their peace and comfort as death nears.

The person may communicate with symbolic gestures, such as reaching upward or toward the ceiling or focusing on something not visible to you. This is not uncommon. There may be times when the dying needs permission to leave or be re-assured that it is OK for them to go. It is

233

most important to always be honest and truthful in any communication. It is OK to tell them how hard it may be to go on without them, but reassuring them you will do your best may be all they need to hear. Communication that conveys a need to keep them here when there is little hope they will not die can bring distress. The hospice team can help if this becomes a stressor for the family. Tears are not a sign of weakness and may be a sign of the love that has existed in the relationship with the person.

Care Includes: Never try to change the perception of what is happening with the person. Provide calm reassurance with your presence and words as you are comfortable. Using cell phones to connect with relatives or important people who live a distance away can provide great comfort to the person. It is important to not argue or try to explain away any visions or conversations they may be having with those who are not present and visible to those present. Most often, these visions or conversations are comforting and can be full of profound meaning to the dying person. If comfortable and it seems appropriate, asking them to share or tell you more might bring insight into what they are experiencing.

In their end-of-life journey, it is important to remember that the pattern of a person's life typically does not change just because they have received a terminal diagnosis and the end of their life is in the foreseeable future. If the

234

person has always been private, outgoing, social, or even humorous, that generally does not change. It is their journey, and we honor them best by following their lead. Wherever that may take us, it is most important to always be honest in your communication with them. Never lie or distort the truth. But convey whatever the truth is with compassion and kindness and be sensitive to what the person desires to know. Offer and explain options or choices for care, but do not expect them to accept what is offered. It is their life, and one of the greatest gifts they can be given is to remain in control of what happens to them. Allowing them to decide is one way of giving them the dignity to continue their life on their terms. They have a right to know all the options available to them, but it is not up to us to direct them to do what we might believe to be in their best interest. Don't try to change them, but help them understand all the possibilities and options by giving information and explanation according to their ability to understand and allowing them the support and encouragement they need to make the choices that work best for them. This is an important way to help them right up to the very end of their life. It is the best way to honor them with dignity as a valuable living human being through their last breath.

Vital Signs and Other Aspects of Comfort

There are many physiologic changes that occur at the

end of life, including muscle weakness, dysphagia, and an altered level of consciousness. Physiologic changes also occur in vital signs such as heart rate, blood pressure, respiratory rate, oxygen saturation, and temperature. Noted changes include increased but weakened heart rate and a drop in blood pressure. The person who has been on blood pressure medications may no longer need these medications. A person who has been on medications such as insulin to manage their blood sugars may no longer need those medications. Looking at the long-range picture, elevated blood sugars no longer carry the detrimental effects they might have early in someone's life. Having an insulin reaction could be a potential problem.

As the body begins to slow and muscles weaken, sphincters become less efficient, and reflexes become sluggish or absent. It is not uncommon that there is a loss of bowel and bladder control. With a decreased intake of food and fluids, bowel movements may decrease but do not stop completely as the body continues to produce secretions to propel contents through the GI tract. Urine can become darker as it is more concentrated with decreased fluid intake.

Marked changes in vital signs often signal cardiovascular instability and/or respiratory compromise and are part of the process of the body shutting down and preparing for death. One of the most observable changes that occurs is the pattern of breathing. Changes in respiratory rate, depth, and oxygen saturation can be noted, as well as apnea (pauses or cessation of breaths) and Cheyne-Stokes respirations (a pattern of breathing that is irregular and sometimes referred to as "agonal breathing"). During Cheyne-Stokes respirations, breathing often occurs in cycles starting with deep and increased respirations that taper in a decreasing pattern followed by pauses (apnea) which can seem lengthy (up to 30 – 60 seconds or longer), and then breathing may resume with deep gasping respirations. This pattern of breathing is not typically distressing to the patient.

The patient may report feeling short of breath, also referred to as air hunger. Shortness of breath is subjective. Oxygen Saturations (SATs – the measure of the blood's oxygen level – normal level would be in the upper 90's to 100%) are not always accurate in assessing a patient's true air hunger. It is better to rely on the person's perception of air hunger. Oxygen is an option, but narcotics and other medications can be effective in relieving the symptoms of shortness of breath as well.

It is also common for the person to have a diminished cough reflex and inability to effectively cough and expectorate secretions or clear the throat. The process of swallowing slows and is compromised. The body produces saliva 24/7, whether the person is alert or unresponsive.

Excess secretions tend to accumulate and can cause congestion. Because the body has a diminished ability to cough and clear away excess secretions, they accumulate and can cause congestion, sometimes referred to as the "death rattle". Extra IV fluids at the end of life can be a source of increased congestion. There are medications available to help dry up or decrease the production of secretions.

Body temperature can also become erratic. The person may appear to be feverish, but it is not typically due to infection. Rather, the temperature-regulating system in the brain is no longer effective or efficient.

The sense of hearing is believed to be the last sense to leave the body. Even though someone may have been hard of hearing or had hearing aids, the sense of hearing seems to remain fully intact to the end. Whatever is said in their presence, even if they seem to be unresponsive, is believed to be heard by the person. It is good to avoid conversations you might not want the person to hear or could be distressing to them.

Care Includes: The patient's comfort remains the most important factor as these changes are happening, and care is directed at what will provide comfort for the patient. There may be no concern for blood pressure or heart rate as they typically don't cause distressing symptoms. Breathing comfort is best effected by keeping the head of the bed slightly elevated, turning the head from side to side as comfortable, and using medications to dry up or decrease the production of secretions. The use of suction is not generally recommended for excessive secretions, as irritation from the suction tip can cause an increase in the production of secretions. Using an oral swab to gently wipe or remove the secretions from the oral cavity are more effective. Air movement using a fan or open window can also be of some benefit. Light covers and air movement also prove beneficial when there is evidence of elevated temperature. A cool cloth on the forehead or back of the neck can be of help, but its benefits are individual and controversial.

Allowing time for each family member to have private time with their loved one, whether it is sharing memories, offering thanks or forgiveness, or just quiet time alone together, can be beneficial and provide a sense of peace for each person. Some people feel the need to share something or talk, or simple touch may be meaningful. Even a simple, quiet presence speaks volumes to the dying person.

Pain and Medications

It is imperative to control pain and any distressing symptoms of terminal illness to allow someone to live out their full potential in life, morally, spiritually, socially, and ethically.

There are many kinds of pain. Physical pain, mental pain, emotional pain from strained relationships, and even spiritual pain have been noted. Physical pain can be of different origins and presents with different sensations as dull, sharp, intense, stabbing, constant, or intermittent. Mental pain can also be from different sources. Mental pain can be the cause of terminal restlessness. Mental pain has the effect of the mind racing in an effort to resolve some real or perceived conflict. As the mind races, the body follows and can exhibit distress with movement or activity that can appear to be unresolved or unsatisfied.

One of the most obvious indications of discomfort from a patient is verbal. Vocalizing discomfort by calling out, moaning, groaning, or other audible indications of discomfort or distress are easily noted. Verbal indications of discomfort, especially with care, turning, or other activities, can easily be addressed. Analgesics can be administered prior to such activities. Discomfort can also be noted in irritability or restlessness, change in muscle tone, and constantly shifting position. Guarding of a painful area, writhing, including grimacing and agitated facial expressions, can be noted.

Nonverbal indications of discomfort can be assessed through what is referred to as a Window of Comfort. If you were to take your hands and frame the face as if you were looking through a window at the person, you could identify discomfort by signs of pain that would include wincing, a furrowed brow, tightened facial muscles, tight closure of eyes and raised cheeks, or an agitated facial expression. If facial muscles are relaxed with no facial grimacing, there is no furrowed brow or tension noted in the face, and the hands are relaxed, and fingers loose with no indication of clenched fists, this would indicate comfort.

A variety of tools are available to assess pain in older adults with advanced dementia. One validated scale commonly used is the Pain Assessment in Advanced Dementia (PAINAD) instrument. Each item is ranked on a scale of 0 to 2, and total scores range from 0 to 10. Higher scores indicate more severe pain (0=no pain and 10=severe pain).

Care Includes: Medications are prioritized upon admission and ongoing. With ongoing decline in status, medications may be changed to crushed if still swallowing safely, or as the disease progresses, they may be discontinued. Eventually, as swallowing becomes difficult or compromised with increased risk for aspiration, medications essential for comfort may be administered in the form of concentrated liquid SL (sub-lingual – under the tongue). Many of the medications used for comfort start to decrease in effectiveness at around four hours. Giving essential comfort medications at four-hour intervals around the clock allows for a maintained therapeutic level of medication in the blood without the peaks and valleys of intermittent dosing. SL medications can easily be administered when the patient is less responsive or unresponsive. It is important to swab the mouth before administration, maintain the HOB (head of the bed) in an elevated position, and support the back of the head and not hyper-extended to prevent aspiration. SL medications are absorbed in the mouth or oral cavity and must be given with care for aspiration.

Medications may be administered in topical cream form, transdermal patches (medication is applied and absorbed through the skin), or rectal suppository routes are also effective and may be indicated. There are many effective ways to administer medication to someone unresponsive. These measures will be helpful in maintaining comfort for the patient. The hospice care team is essential in planning timing of medications essential for comfort and the best method of administration.

The above-mentioned measures will be helpful in maintaining comfort for the patient. If the patient is comfortable, the family will also experience less distress during this challenging time.

A rule of thumb with medications for whatever reason they are administered is to start low and go slow when increasing the dosage. It is also important to remember that any of the above-mentioned signs or symptoms may or may not occur with your loved one. Everyone is unique in their life. Whatever is happening or whatever symptoms appear, it is always important to share this information with the hospice care team, who can effectively provide information and the management of those symptoms. Hospice caregivers are experts in End of Life care. "On call" staff are available 24/7 and should be consulted with any questions or concerns that may arise. No one, patient or family, needs to walk this journey alone.

Any fact facing us is not as important as our attitude toward it, for that determines our success or failure.

- Norman Vincent Peale

-

"And what is as important as knowledge?" asked the mind.

"Seeing and caring with the heart," answered the soul.

- Flavia Weedn

Part IV: Spirituality

Death is more than just a physical process. The spirit and the body are inescapably involved in life's final reckoning. Every dying process includes a spiritual dimension. Something more than the physiological closing down of the body's systems happens as death approaches. It is not uncommon that dying people often feel compelled to confront and resolve unfinished issues from their past. There may be issues with former relationships, family members, or even spiritual issues that need to be addressed. The reality of the nearness of death can awaken a powerful appreciation for the wonder and mystery of life itself. Human beings are inherently built in such a way that they find the most value in those things which are finite. There are many sacred moments that occur in the last intimate days of a person's life. Hospice workers and family become witnesses to the awe that occurs in the extraordinary acts of love, trust and courage, acceptance and forgiveness. Those working in hospice are privileged to be witness to much holiness and beauty.

The holistic approach by hospice addresses any issues or concerns that may need some resolution for a patient. Spiritual needs often surface, and hospice provides support in whatever faith tradition the patient desires or requests. It may mean notifying their preferred local religious community or helping someone reconnect with a faith community they may have been away from for some time. A Spiritual Care Coordinator is available for support for any spiritual concerns or issues. If a person has no desire for a spiritual connection, that is honored. A person may not feel comfortable reconnecting with a former faith community but may feel the need for some type of spiritual support. Hospice will offer support in any way the patient needs but does not force or pressure anyone. It is the patient's journey, and their wishes are honored and respected.

Spirituality is the deep inner essence of who we are. Spirituality can be the music that plays in the background of our lives, providing guidance, direction, reassurance, and hope for the future. Related to our soul, spirituality comes from the unique qualities of each individual. It is the deeply held convictions and feelings with respect to life's meaning and purpose. It can include religious practices which externally express one's interior beliefs. Spirituality and religion can ideally enhance the final stage of life. Spirituality is based on personal experiences and relationship with God, nature, or a higher power. Spirituality can help people find hope when in the midst of despair. Spiritual issues are central in life and particularly at the end of life. Spirituality is found in all cultures and societies and is expressed in an individual's search for ultimate meaning. In the holistic approach to care by hospice, patients are more satisfied because the whole person (body, mind, and spirit) is treated and not just the illness or disease. Treatments and care are enhanced when conversations center around the person's values and beliefs.

There are times in all our lives when we are forced to reach deep into the core of our being to find what is the truth of our real nature. What do I know most deeply to be true? Who do I believe myself to be? What have I placed at the center of my life? Where do I belong, and what will people find as the legacy of my life when it is over? What has been my gift to the family of humanity?

When faced with terminal illness and end of life, these questions can become paramount to the person. Oftentimes we find patients reprioritizing their lives where they can find a deep sense of meaning and purpose in the knowledge that life's days are numbered. There is no better classroom about the bedrock truths of life than the deathbed. It is there we find that we are fragile human beings who are here for only a short time. Throughout life, we may have lost some perspective about these important issues of life, but the dying often find what is most important in life is love, compassion, and human connection.

When illness occurs, many people turn inward to

understand and deal with the crisis. They ask questions like: "Why is this happening to me?" "What is my purpose in this life?" "What will happen to me when life ends?" Serious illness frequently causes one to reflect on what it is that really matters in life. As life is coming to an end and the body is becoming more frail, it is not uncommon that the individual's inner being becomes stronger as their deep and maybe hidden spirituality is awakened. As death approaches, it is not uncommon that spiritual concerns become even more important. This re-appraisal of one's life can bring about many positive changes. Priorities might change, and a person's entire outlook on life may change.

A traditional way that spirituality has been expressed throughout the ages is through the medium of story. Through story, both oral and written, sacred people, places, and events are preserved. Some of the universal aspects of spirituality are addressed through a review of one's life.

"Has my life been worthwhile?" is a common question asked by seriously ill people who are trying to find out whether they have made an impact on the lives of others close to them and society as a whole. Doing a life review — looking at photographs, watching movies, or listening to music from particular periods — allows the person to reminisce about events and relationships throughout their life. It can help them rediscover legacies, meaning, and spiritual strengths. It may be possible for the dying to recognize the divine within their unique life experience. It is important to allow people to tell their sacred stories and, in the telling, may reveal underlying truths, teachings, and the meaning that life presents. Each person's life story is a book of its own which may reveal much wisdom and understanding. The mere gift of listening to the stories can bring relief to the dying as they reminisce about their life experiences. A compassionate listening presence can make a big difference for the dying. Stories help us to make sense of our lives. When an individual dies and is buried, the library of their life is buried with them.

Terminally ill persons can die meaningfully in a way that is consistent with their own identity. Because death is a personal experience, each person will define his or her own appropriate death differently. As part of this process, a terminally ill person may seek to feel connected to others. This may lead to maintaining and deepening existing relationships, putting affairs in order, and taking care of unfinished business.

Another spiritual need is transcendence, or a person's awareness and acknowledgment of issues that transcend, or go beyond, earthly concerns. Each person may want assurance that, in some way, life will continue after death occurs. Some may turn to God for guidance and comfort, while others may focus on the legacy they leave behind.

Being alert to things that may indicate a person is experiencing a loss of meaning or purpose may be found in comments like "I am so alone, or I feel hopeless; what's the point." "I don't know who I am anymore", "I don't want to be a burden," or "I need to make amends." The person may not verbalize their specific concerns, so it's important to be aware of their behavior and actions. For example, they may seem afraid of being alone or refuse help when they appear to need it. It is not uncommon for those who are facing the end of life to wonder if there is life after death. This can be a deeply spiritual concern, along with wondering whether one's life has had meaning or purpose.

A sick man turned to his doctor as he was preparing to leave the examination room. He turned and said, "Doctor, I am afraid to die. Tell me what lies on the other side." Very quietly, the doctor said, "I don't know." "You don't know? You, a Christian man, do not know what is on the other side?"

The doctor was holding the handle of the door; on the other side came a sound of scratching and whining, and as he opened the door, a dog sprang into the room and leaped on him with an eager show of gladness. Turning to the patient, the doctor said, "Did you notice my dog? He's never been in this room before. He didn't know what was inside. He knew nothing except that his master was here, and when the door opened, he sprang in without fear. I know little of what is on the other side of death, but I do know one thing...I know my Master is there, and that is enough."

The final stage of life offers the possibility of healing relationships, healing feelings of regret and guilt, and offering love and forgiveness where needed. Many kinds of healing can still unfold even when healing of the body is no longer a possibility.

One of the most important things to do is listen without judgment or dismissing what the person is saying. Try to understand and accommodate the patient's beliefs without imposing your own. If the person is thinking about worries from the past, encouraging them to talk about good memories may help. If they're anxious or afraid, try to understand what they're worried about. For example, some people are afraid of the pain becoming too much or being alone when they die. If it seems appropriate, holding hands or a hug with the person's approval may be reassuring. Always ask for permission.

Questions about life and its meaning are profound, so don't feel like there always needs to be an answer. Leave room for attentive listening, thoughtfulness, reflection, and stillness. The ministry of presence cannot be overstated. Just being present speaks volumes to the dying. It is important to help the patient maintain hope and find strength in trusting others as they search for meaning and maintain a sense of purpose in the life they live. It is important to comfort those we cannot cure. Hospice is about helping people die with dignity and live out life with love.

Ira Byock, M.D., is a leading palliative care physician and long-time public advocate for improving care through the end of life. In his book, "The Four Things That Matter Most", he offers us four simple life-affirming phrases "Please forgive me", "I forgive you", "Thank you", and "I love you". These four simple phrases carry enormous power, and in many ways, they contain the most powerful words in our language. The stories in this book show us that emotional healing is always possible, even in the wake of family strife, personal tragedy, divorce, and even in the face of death.

Life is like a tapestry. We see the finished needlepoint from above that looks so beautiful. But we seldom see the underside with the chaos of strands of thread that seem to have no purpose. But the weaving of all the colors, dark and bright, are woven together to make for the best piece possible. Life is like that. That which goes into making it beautiful may not always look appealing or with purpose, as the underside of the tapestry. But the finished product is exactly what it was intended to be. And all of it was necessary for it to be complete.

Tapestry Poem

My life is but a weaving

Between my God and me.

I cannot choose the colors

He weaveth steadily.

Oft 'times He weaveth sorrow;

And I, in foolish pride

Forget He sees the upper

And I the underside.

Not 'til the loom is silent

And the shuttles cease to fly

Will God unroll the canvas

And reveal the reason why.

The dark threads are as needful

In the weaver's skillful hand

As the threads of gold and silver

In the pattern He has planned

He knows, He loves, He cares;

Nothing this truth can dim.

He gives the very best to those

Who leave the choice to Him.

– Author Unknown –

Often quoted by Corrie ten Boom

Loss and Survival Strategies

Every stage of life has its own challenges and opportunities. As human beings, we experience an underlying theme of letting go throughout our life. If a tiny baby in the womb were aware of what's ahead through the process of labor and delivery, it would be afraid of birth. If there were a choice, the baby would probably decline to go through the process. To leave the only world it has known would seem like a kind of death. But immediately after birth, the infant would find itself in loving arms, showered with affection, and cared for at every moment. Surely, the baby would say, "I was foolish to doubt God's plan for me. This is a beautiful place to be."

Death is as predictable a part of living as being born and growing. It is said that growth is painful (i.e., growing pains). Losing someone you love or care deeply about is one of the most painful experiences in life. But there is also a potential for growth in spite of the heartache of loss. The more significant the loss, the more intense the grief. Grief is the emotional suffering one feels when something or someone you love is taken away. Even subtle losses can lead to grief. The outward expression of grief is called mourning. The acute phase happens shortly after a loss is experienced and can last for different amounts of time. Symptoms of acute grief can range from sadness to an intense longing for and thoughts of the person who has died. Anxiety, anger, and crying are expressions of mourning. Grief can turn our world upside down. It cannot be "fixed," and we should not try to fix it. Our mourning speaks loudly, "Something important happened to me. I am hurting; I feel lost and broken".

Grief never ends because our love never ends. We are not supposed to "get over it" because we can never get over the love we shared with the person who died. The feelings of loss never completely disappear, but the intense feelings will soften, and the deep pain of grief does lessen with time. The sadness and acute symptoms of grief we experience following a deep loss force us to slow down. The ritual of having a wake and funeral are all intentional to help us slow down and acknowledge what has happened and regroup and consider what to do next. Throughout history, important events or transitions in life that are profound have brought us back to ritual to know what to do. Think of birth, graduations, weddings, and even death and funerals. We look to traditions and rituals to help us know how to honor and respect these holy moments in life.

Grief and mourning are essential parts of the healing process needed following a great loss. We love from the outside in, and we grieve from the inside out. All grief is very personal and individual. The grieving process takes time. Healing happens gradually and cannot be forced or

255

hurried. There is no "normal" timetable for grieving. And there is no right or wrong way to grieve. David Kessler, noted grief specialist, states that grief is like snowflakes and fingerprints. No two are alike, and all are unique to the person.

There are healthy ways to cope with the pain that, in time, can renew us and help us move on. In 1969, psychiatrist Elisabeth Kubler-Ross introduced what became known as the "five stages of grief". These stages of grief were based on her studies of the feelings of patients facing terminal illnesses. She never intended the stages to be a roadmap through grief. The five stages are Denial, "This can't be happening to me", Anger, "Why is this happening? Who is to blame?" Bargaining, "Make this not happen, and in return, I will _____", Depression, "I'm too sad to do anything", and Acceptance," I'm at peace with what happened." These stages are a guide and offer some understanding of the many emotions of someone who is grieving. Not everyone who grieves goes through each of the stages, and they are not linear, happening in a sequence.

Kubler-Ross never intended for these stages to be a rigid framework that applies to everyone who grieves. In her last book before her death in 2004, she said of the five stages: "They were never meant to help tuck messy emotions into neat packages. They are responses to loss that many people have, but there is not a typical response to loss as there is no typical loss. "Loving someone changes us forever. And so does losing them." Finding support from family or friends who understand without expecting a certain outcome is helpful. Support groups where one can share their sorrow and feel they are being heard in their grief are valuable resources. Drawing comfort from one's faith tradition can offer solace, as well as journaling your thoughts and feelings.

It's important to take care of yourself and express your true feelings in a safe environment, wherever you find that safe place. It is normal to feel sad, numb, or angry following a loss. As time passes, these emotions should become less intense. If you aren't accepting the loss and starting to move forward, feeling better over time, or grief seems to be getting worse, it may be the grief has become complicated. When this happens, it is recommended to reach out for professional help. There is nothing wrong with asking for additional help. It is a very healthy and constructive way to find your way forward.

After the deep loss experienced by a young child who was asked if he thought things might be getting better, he responded, "No, mom, they're just less worse!" An older adolescent responded similarly by saying, "We've come a long way; we just haven't gotten very far." These are innocent but very true statements. It takes time and support, which can come in many ways. As Megan McKenna noted in her book "And Morning Came", we are challenged to "make music out of what remains of our lives, our loves, our dreams, our hopes and fears, our sufferings, our struggles, our relationships, and faithfulness."

It is a time to live life by striking a line through every minus, turning it into a plus. The Dalai Lama tells us, "Our prime purpose in this life is to help others. And if you can't help them, at least just don't hurt them." The very process of grief renders one vulnerable and more fully human. Grief is a time of personal reflection during which we assess the very meaning of our existence. C.S. Lewis states, "Grief is like a long winding valley where any bend may reveal a totally new landscape."

Whether it is accompanying the person who has just received the diagnosis of a terminal illness, or someone who has just experienced the devastating loss of a loved one, showing kindness, empathy, and understanding or just being considerate of the situation can help alleviate some of the turmoil surrounding the life-changing situation. Kindness generates the human bond of caring, compassion, and empathy. The value of kindness derives from connection, bonding, and kinship with another human being. Simply being there and walking side by side on the painful journey speaks volumes to the person suffering the loss. We don't walk in front trying to lead them or follow behind, helping to pick up the pieces, but we walk side by side, carrying them when needed with the love we have for them.

This kindness flows from empathy, embracing, and making a connection with the feelings of another. Kindness and compassion are not about changing the situation to help us feel comfortable. It is about being on the journey and being there in the fire of the moment. Being on the journey with a loved one is about assuring them they will not be abandoned no matter what happens, and we will face whatever comes together. When the going gets tough, when others decide they need to step out or away, the true friend with empathy becomes the steady presence that says you are important, and this matters.

"Who, then, can so softly bind up the wound of another as he who has felt the same wound?"

- Thomas Jefferson

Part V: Epilogue

Writing this book has been a dream of mine for a very long time. My first love in nursing was working in the Obstetrics department, where birth and new life on earth begins. Then I was privileged to work in the setting of chronic illness where people faced life-long disease and illness that impacts all of life. Having worked in hospice care the remaining years of my nursing career seems to have completed the circle of life for me from a nursing perspective. Every aspect of nursing is important, and I feel privileged to have had this unique combination of experiences in health care where each opportunity has taught me great things beyond the medical experience. I have learned about life, coping, the challenges in health, loss, and most importantly, the true reason for all existence. That is to be here and accompany those who face these challenges and offer the support and knowledge that can help to make this mysterious journey of life less fearful, threatening, and painful. We are all here to help one another, and it is the most important job assigned to any of us.

Having worked with the best healthcare professionals who work with caring and loving hearts has been a privilege. Working with patients who face challenges daily, and who consistently step up with courage, trust, and hope has been most inspiring. No one knows what tomorrow will bring, but having people beside you to walk with you on a journey that seems to have no roadmap or, at times, direction, brings much perspective to life. It is all about the love, caring, compassion, and courage that it takes every day to make it a good one. And each of us makes choices daily about what our life will be like. I am grateful for the many people who have influenced me, who have allowed me to be part of their journey, who have trusted me, and who have journeyed with me along this path of my life. I could not have done it without any one of them. They have all been the best gifts to me.

When I started writing this book, my intention was to help all who read it realize that life has many stages and there is always a beginning and an end. There can be joy and meaning at every turn. And there are always those who are willing to help us along the way. I also wanted to help people know that having the support of hospice care does not necessarily mean "this is the end." There is much life to be lived at every turn and at every moment. And there can be meaning, purpose, hope, and love every step of the way. Even in the last moments of life, there can be so much more than just an end. It is important to cherish every moment, and even in loss, there is much to be learned.

I hope you have enjoyed the stories, and I invite you to

share your story with others. Every story has meaning and is important. I ask God's blessing on all who read this, and I wish for you beautiful moments and beautiful music as you continue on this mysterious but wonder-filled journey of life.

"You matter because you are you, and you matter to the end of your life. We will do all we can, not only to help you die peacefully but also to live until you die."

- Dame Cicely Saunders, founder of the modern Hospice Movement

Part VI: Selected Bibliography and Further Reading

What the Dying Have to Teach Us - Medicine and What Matters in the End - Grief & Loss

Albom, Mitch. Tuesdays With Morrie: An Old Man, A Young Man, and Life's Greatest Lesson. New York: Doubleday, 1997.

Alexander, Even, MD. Proof of Heaven. New York: Simon & Schuster, 2012.

Amatuzio, Janis, MD. Beyond Knowing: Mysteries & Messages of Death & Life from a Forensic Pathologist. Novato, CA: New World Library, 2006.

Amatuzio, Janis, MD. Forever Ours: Real Stories of Immortality and Living from a Forensic Pathologist. Novato, CA: New World Library, 2002.

Back, Anthony and Arnold, Robert. Mastering Communication with Seriously Ill Patients: Balancing Honest with Empathy and Hope. Cambridge, England: Cambridge University Press, 2010.

Baines, Barry K., MD. Ethical Wills: Putting Your Values on Paper. Cambridge, MA: Perseus Publishing, 2002.

Byock, Ira, MD. Dying Well: Peace and Possibilities at the

End of Life. New York: Riverhead Books, 1997.

Byock, Ira, MD. The Best Care Possible: A Physician's Quest to Transform Care Through End of Life. New York: Avery-Penguin Group, 2012.

Byock, Ira, MD. The Four Things That Matter Most: A Book About Living. New York: Free Press, 2004.

Callahan, Daniel. The Troubled Dream of Life: Living Mortality. New York: Simon & Schuster, 1993.

Callanan, Maggie. Final Journeys. New York: Bantam Books, 2008.

Callanan, Maggie and Kelly, Patricia. Final Gifts. New York: Bantam Books, 1993.

Davis, Verdell. Let Me Grieve But Not Forever, A Journey Out of the Darkness of Loss. Dallas: Word Publishing Group, 1994.

DeHennezel, Marie. Intimate Death: How the Dying Teach Us to Live. London, England: Abacus Publishing, 2001.

Dowling Singh, Kathleen. The Grace in Dying: A Message of Hope, Comfort and Spiritual Transformation. San Francisco, CA: Harper One, 2000.

Edwards, Deanna. Grieving, The Pain and the Promise. Covenant Communications, American Fork, Utah: 1989

Gutkind, Lee. At the End of Life: True Stories About How

We Die. Pittsburgh, PA: Creative Non-Fiction, 2011.

Gutkind, Lee. Twelve Breath A Minute: End of Life Essays. Dallas, TX: Southern Methodist University Press, 2011.

Gawande, Atul, MD. Being Mortal. New York: Metropolitan Books, 2014.

Gawande, Atul, MD. Better: A Surgeon's Notes on Performance. New York: Metropolitan Books, 2007.

Gawande, Atul, MD. The Checklist Manifesto: How to Get Things Right. New York: Picador, 2010.

Hutchison, Joyce, RN, and Rupp, Joyce. May I Walk You Home? Courage and Comfort for Caregivers of the Very Ill. Notre Dame, IN: Ave Maria Press, 1999.

Kalanithi, Paul. When Breath Becomes Air. New York: Random House, 2016.

Karnes, Barbara, RN. Gone From My Sight. Vancouver: Barbara Karnes, 1986.

Kearney, Micheal, MD. Mortally Wounded: Stories of Soul Pain, Death, and Healing. New York: Touchstone Books, 1997.

Kessler, David. The Needs of the Dying: A Guide for Bringing Hope, Comfort and Love to Life's Final Chapter. New York: Harper Collins, 1997.

Kessler, David. Visions, Trips and Crowded Rooms: Who

and What You See Before You Die. Carlsbad, CA: Hay House, 2010.

Kubler-Ross, Elisabeth, MD. Death, The Final Stage of Growth. Englewood Cliffs, NJ: Prentice Hall, Inc., 1975

Kubler-Ross, Elisabeth, MD. Living with Death and Dying. New York: McMillan Publishing, 1981.

Kubler-Ross, Elisabeth, MD. On Children and Death: How Children and their Parents Can and Do Cope with Death. New York: Touchstone, 1983.

Kubler-Ross, Elisabeth, MD. On Death and Dying: What the Dying have to Teach Doctors, Nurses, Clergy, and their own Families. New York: Scribner, 1969.

Kubler-Ross, Elisabeth, MD. On Life After Death. Berkeley, CA: Celestial Arts, 1991.

Kubler-Ross, Elisabeth, MD. The Tunnel and the Light: Essential Insights on Living and Dying. New York: Marlowe & Company, 1999.

Kubler-Ross, Elisabeth, MD. The Wheel of Life: A Memoir of Living and Dying. New York: Touchstone, 1997.

Kubler-Ross, Elisabeth, MD and Kessler, David. Life Lessons: Two Experts on Death and Dying Teach Us About the Mysteries of Life and Living. New York: Touchstone, 2000.

Kubler-Ross, Elisabeth, MD and Kessler, David. On Grief

and Grieving, Finding Meaning of Grief Through the Five Stages of Loss. New York: Scribner, 2005.

Lynn, Joanne, MD and Harrold, Joan, MD. Handbook for Mortals: Guidance for People Facing Serious Illness. New York: Oxford University Press, 1999.

MacGregor, Betsy, MD. In Awe of Being Human: A Doctor's Stores from the Edge of Life and Death. Greenbank, WA: Abiding Nowhere Press, 2013.

McKenna, Megan. And Morning Came: Scriptures of the Resurrection. Lanham, MD: Sheed & Ward, 2003.

Metzgar, Margaret K., M.A. LMHC, et. al. A Time to Mourn, A Time to Dance: Help for the Losses in Life. Appleton, WI: Thrivent Financial for Lutherans, 2006.

Miller, Glen E. Living Thoughtfully, Dying Well: A Doctor Explains How to Make Death A Natural Part of Life. Harrisonburg, VA: Herald Press, 2014.

Moreland Jones, Doris. And Not One Bird Stopped Singing, Coping with Transition and Loss in Aging. Nashville, TN: Upper Room Books, 1997.

Noel, Brook and Blair, Pamela D, Ph.D. I Wasn't Ready to Say Goodbye: Surviving, Coping & Healing after the Sudden Death of a Loved One. Naperville, IL: Source Books Inc., 2000.

Nuland, Sherwin B. How We Die: Reflections on Life's

Final Chapter. New York: Vintage Books, 1993.

Olsen, Melody, Ph.D., RN. Healing the Dying. Albany, NY: Delmar Publishers, 2001.

Pausch, Randy and Zaslow, Jeffrey. The Last Lecture. New York: Hyperion, 2008.

Preston, Thomas A, MD. Final Victory: Taking Charge of The Last Stages of Life, Facing Death on Your Own Terms. Roseville, CA: Forum Press, 2000.

Remen, Rachel Namoi, MD. Kitchen Table Wisdom, Stories That Heal. New York: Riverhead Books, 1996.

Siegal, Bernie S., MD. Love Medicine & Miracles. New York: Harper & Row Publisher, 1986.

Siegal, Bernie S., MD. Peace, Love & Healing. New York: Harper & Row, 1989.

Simmons, Philip. Learning to Fall: The Blessings of an Imperfect Life. New York: Bantam Books, 2000.

Smith, Doug and Pittman, Marilu. The TAO of Dying: A Guide to Caring. Washington, DC: Caring Publishers, 1997.

Volandes, Angelo MD. The Conversation: A Revolutionary Plan for End of Life Care. New York: Bloomsbury, 2015.

Weisse, Allen B., MD. Lessons in Mortality, Doctors and Patients Struggling Together. Columbia, MO: University of Missouri Press, 2006.

Warraich, Haider, MD. Modern Death, How Medicine Changed the End of Life. New York: St. Martins Press, 2017.

Wolfelt, Alan D., PhD. Healing the Adult Child's Grieving Heart: 100 Practical Ideas After Your Parent Dies. Ft. Collins, CO: Companion Press, 2002.

Along with the above named books, there are numerous websites and organizations that support and encourage education and understanding about the end of life choices and care, loss, and grief.

https://www.nhpco.org/

https://agingwithdignity.org/

https://fivewishes.org/Home

http://gowish.org/

www.ingramcontent.com/pod-product-compliance
Lightning Source LLC
Chambersburg PA
CBHW040847210326
41597CB00029B/4760